CONTENTS

Acknowledgments

I would like to express my sincere thanks and appreciation to many people and drug companies for helping me complete this material: to the Essex Community College for making this project possible; to Rhoda Levin, Dr. Lois Linn, Arianne Regester, and Eleanor Greentree of Essex Community College; to my other colleagues at Essex Community College for their help and encouragement; to Dot Pope, Deborah Zink and Ruth Wright for typing the manuscript; to Roger Heer, Director of Pharmacy, Franklin Square Hospital, Baltimore County, Maryland; to Michael Ledrick, Staff Pharmacist, Franklin Square Hospital for help with the Pediatric Dosage unit; to the following drug companies for the use of their copyrighted drug labels:—Eli Lilly and Company; Bristol Laboratories; Parke-Davis; Smith Kline & French Laboratories*; Abbott Laboratories; Merck Sharp and Dohme, Pfizer Laboratories Division; and to all others who have helped in any way.

*All Labels are current as of November, 1980.

To my Husband, Charles.

PREFACE

In 1972, I began to write teaching units in dosage and solutions problems for use in my Nursing classes at the Essex Community College. As I worked with students, some of whom suffered from "math anxiety", I saw the need for a textbook in the calculation of dosages that was clear and concise, written in a manner in which the principles and problems of dosages and solutions might be simply stated, without compromising either the necessary information, or insulting the intelligence of the Nursing student. I wanted a book that was student rather than teacher oriented.

In 1978, I received a grant from the Division of Allied Health of the Essex Community College, Baltimore County, Maryland to prepare such a workbook. The essentials of this book were completed in the Summer of 1978. Since then, on the basis of suggestions offered by my students and colleagues, I have subjected this text to annual review, revision, and expansion. Through the years, this book has been used as a selfstudy text for Nursing students. It has also been employed in the classroom as a textbook for Nursing students, and for Registered Nurses wishing to return to practice after years of absence from the field. In addition, this book has been used as a text in two classes which I conducted for Graduate Nurses who, although active in the profession, wished to sharpen their skills in preparing dosages and solutions.

This book is practice oriented. It makes use of drug labels, syringes, and medicine glasses in an attempt to make the exercises relevant to actual Nursing practice. Throughout, the emphasis is placed upon the metric system of measurements. However, ample attention is devoted to the apothecaries' system. Metric-apothecaries' conversion exercises are included for the benefit of those nurses who serve where drugs are still ordered in apothecaries' units. The workbook treats intravenous flow rate in a simplified manner. The Pediatric Dosage unit includes the traditional formulas, but adds body surface area calculations, and dosages per body weight calculations. There is a unit in reading drug labels. Exercises are included in reconstituting powdered drugs using actual drug labels. The use of the 24-hour clock in new computer patient drug print-outs, the "kardex" of the future, is explained.

It is in the belief that this workbook, born out of my pedagogical frustrations, developed in my classroom, and tested, expanded, and confirmed in my teaching experience will meet the needs of instructors, students, and Registered Nurses, that I offer this work to my colleagues in the Nursing–Teaching professions.

Mary Ann Fravel Norville

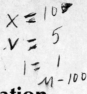

Arithmetic Self-Evaluation

The number concepts needed to master the content of this dosage workbook are exemplified in the following problems. Work each set of examples to see if you remember how to find the answer. The explanations and answers will be found on the pages following the test.

1. Circle the largest number in each set. Underline the smallest number.
   a. 1/4, 4/8, 3/16
   b. 8/9, 8/25, 8/125
   c. 0.5, 0.25, 0.125
   d. 0.325, 1.3333, 1.75

2. Add the following fractions and mixed numbers.
   a. 7/8 + 5/4 = _____
   b. 10 1/2 + 12 1/4 + 16 3/4 = _____
   c. 3/4 + 1/6 + 1/8 = _____
   d. 7 1/12 + 3 2/3 + 8 5/24 = _____

3. Add the following decimals.
   a. 10.4 + 45.62 + 0.44 = _____
   b. 0.01 + 0.625 + 2.3 = _____
   c. 16 + 8.24 + 0.084 = _____
   d. 0.125 + 0.025 + 0.05 = _____

4. Subtract the following fractions and mixed numbers.
   a. 2/3 − 1/4 = _____
   b. 6 2/5 − 5 3/10 = _____
   c. 100 1/33 − 33 1/3 = _____
   d. 175 4/6 − 148 1/3 = _____

5. Subtract the following decimal fractions.

    a. $950 - 250.25 =$ _____

    b. $0.05 - 0.025 =$ _____

    c. $16.23 - 14.293 =$ _____

    d. $2.8 - 0.95 =$ _____

6. Multiply the following fractions.

    a. $2/4 \times 4/6 =$ _____

    b. $1/2 \times 1/3 =$ _____

    c. $5\ 1/6 \times 1/8 =$ _____

    d. $4\ 4/5 \times 2\ 1/5 \times 8\ 1/4 =$ _____

7. Multiply the following decimals.

    a. $1.5 \times 3 =$ _____

    b. $0.05 \times 1.5 =$ _____

    c. $36.284 \times 7.21 =$ _____

    d. $0.0033 \times 6.02 =$ _____

8. Divide the following fractions.

    a. $1/2 \div 1/3 =$ _____

    b. $1/150 \div 1/2 =$ _____

    c. $3\ 3/4 \div 2/3 =$ _____

    d. $\dfrac{1\ 1/2}{7/8} \div \dfrac{1\ 1/3}{2\ 1/2} =$ _____

9. Divide the following decimals.

    a. $64.5 \div 2.5 =$ _____

    b. $2.5 \div 0.01 =$ _____

    c. $12.075 \div 2.5 =$ _____

    d. $0.065 \div 10 =$ _____

10. Solve for N using a formula.

    a. $\dfrac{24}{48} \times 5 = N$

    b. $\dfrac{120}{60} \times 2.2 = N$

c. $\dfrac{3.5}{1.75} \times 5 = N$

d. $\dfrac{32}{16} \times N = 60$

11. *Solve for X using ratio and proportion.*

    a. $5 : 20 : : 2 : X$

    b. $1/6 : 1 : : X : 1\ 1/2$

    c. $\dfrac{2.5}{X} : : \dfrac{5}{10}$

    d. $\dfrac{X}{3/4} : : \dfrac{7/9}{21/24}$

12. *Write the following Arabic numbers as Román numĕrals.*

    a. 8 _VIII_
    b. 3 _III_
    c. 21 _XX̶I̶ XXI_
    d. 50 _L_

13. *Write the following Roman numerals as Arabic numbers.*

    a. CIV _104_
    b. XL _40_
    c. MCMLXXXI _2/185_
    d. XV _15_

14. *Change the following units to the indicated equivalents.*

	PERCENTAGE	DECIMAL	FRACTION	RATIO
a.	10%	0.10	1/10	1:10
b.	65%	0.65	65/100	
c.	25%	.25	1/4	
d.	0.2%	.3/10	1/500	1:500

Answers: Arithmetic Self-Evaluation

1. *Circle the largest number in each set. Underline the smallest number.*

   a. 1/4, (4/8), 3/16

   $$\underline{\frac{4}{16}} \quad \frac{8}{16} \quad \frac{3}{16}$$

   In order to compare the relative value of each fraction, first find the common denominator for the group of fractions and then compare their value. To help you visualize these concepts, you might also think of these fractions in terms of familiar illustrations from life, for example, as the parts into which three pies are divided. You know that if you are served 1/4 of a pie, the pie has been divided into four parts.

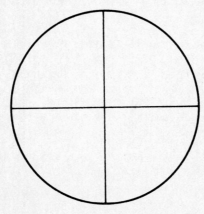

   <u>1</u> The *numerator* tells us how many parts are involved.

   <u>4</u> The *denominator* tells us how many parts are in the whole (in this case, the number of parts into which the pie was divided) and the numerator tells you how many parts you received.

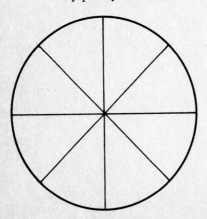

   If the same pie was divided into eight parts, you know each part will be smaller, or 1/2 the size of those in the first pie. Since you will receive 4/8 of the pie, this means you will receive 4 parts of the pie which will equal 1/2 of the pie: $\frac{4}{8} = \frac{1}{2}$.

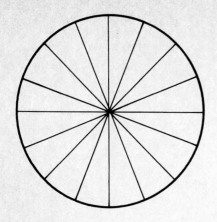

Now if the pie is divided into 16 parts, each part will be only a quarter of the size of those in the first pie. The three parts that you receive do not equal 1/4 of the pie, as in the case of the pie divided into only four parts. You know that this is a smaller fraction.

b. numerator $\left(\dfrac{8}{9}\right)$, $\dfrac{8}{25}$, $\dfrac{8}{125}$
   denominator

The smaller the denominator, the larger the parts that the whole has been divided into. The larger the denominator, the smaller the parts of the whole. The numerators are all the same. In the first fraction, 8/9, you are dealing with 8 parts out of a total of 9 parts. The second fraction is 8 parts out of a total of 25 parts. The third fraction is 8 parts out of a total of 125 parts—a much smaller proportion.

c. $\boxed{0.5}$, 0.25, 0.125

You may think of decimal fractions as 5/10, 25/100, and 125/1,000.

$$\dfrac{5}{10} = \dfrac{1}{2} \qquad \dfrac{25}{100} = \dfrac{1}{4} \qquad \dfrac{125}{1,000} = \dfrac{1}{8}$$

Another familiar example may involve money. 0.5 is the same as 0.50 or 50¢. 0.25 or 25¢ and 0.125 or 12½¢.

d. 0.325, 1.3333, $\boxed{1.75}$

Think fractions $\dfrac{325}{1,000}$, $1\dfrac{3333}{10,000}$, $1\dfrac{75}{100}$

Numbers to the left of a decimal point are whole numbers.

or

Think money   32½¢, $1.33\dfrac{1}{3}$, $1.75

Numbers to the right of a decimal point are fractions of a whole number.

2. *Add the following fractions and mixed numbers.*

a. numerator $\dfrac{7}{8} + \dfrac{5}{4} = \dfrac{7}{8} + \dfrac{10}{8} = \dfrac{17}{8} = 2\dfrac{1}{8}$
   denominator

When adding fractions you must *first* be sure that each fraction has the same denominator. If the denominators are not the same, find a common denominator. (A common denominator is a number into which all of the denominators will devide evenly.) *Next*, you must add the numerators together. In this example, you want to know how many 8ths you have. When added, you have 17 eighths.

Divide 17 by 8 to change the fraction to a mixed number: $\dfrac{17}{8} = 2\dfrac{1}{8}$.

b. $10\dfrac{1}{2} = \dfrac{2}{4}$

$12\dfrac{1}{4} = \dfrac{1}{4}$

$16\dfrac{3}{4} = \dfrac{3}{4}$

$\overline{}$

$38 \qquad \dfrac{6}{4} = 1\dfrac{2}{4} = 1\dfrac{1}{2}$

$1\dfrac{1}{2}$

$\overline{}$

$39\dfrac{1}{2}$

Find a common denominator for the fractions and add the numerators to see how many 4ths you have. You have 6/4 which is an improper fraction. When reduced you have 1 1/2; add this to the number obtained when you added the whole numbers.

c. $\dfrac{3}{4} = \dfrac{18}{24}$

$\dfrac{1}{6} = \dfrac{4}{24}$

$\dfrac{1}{8} = \dfrac{3}{24}$

$\overline{}$

$\dfrac{25}{24} = 1\dfrac{1}{24}$

The least common denominator for 4, 6, and 8 is 24.

d. $7\dfrac{1}{12} = 7\dfrac{2}{24}$

$3\dfrac{2}{3} = 3\dfrac{16}{24}$

$8\dfrac{5}{24} = 8\dfrac{5}{24}$

$\overline{}$

$18\dfrac{23}{24}$

3. *Add the following decimals.*

a.
```
 10.40
 45.62
  0.44
------
 56.46
```

You may add a zero to keep the columns straight. Line up the numbers so the decimal points are in a straight line. Then add the columns as you would whole numbers. Remember to place the decimal point in the answer. It should be placed directly under the other decimal points.

b.
```
0.010
0.625
2.300
-----
2.935
```

c.
```
16.000
 8.240
 0.084
------
24.324
```

d.
```
0.125
0.025
0.050
-----
0.200
```

4. *Subtract the following fractions and mixed numbers.*

a.
$$\frac{2}{3} = \frac{8}{12}$$
$$-\frac{1}{4} = \frac{3}{12}$$
$$\frac{5}{12}$$

Before you can subtract fractions you must find a common denominator.

b.
$$6\frac{2}{5} = 6\frac{4}{10}$$
$$-5\frac{3}{10} = 5\frac{3}{10}$$
$$1\frac{1}{10}$$

c.
$$100\frac{1}{33} = \overset{99}{\cancel{100}}\frac{\overset{33}{+1}}{33} = \frac{34}{33}$$
$$-33\frac{1}{3} = -33\frac{11}{33} = \frac{11}{33}$$
$$66 \qquad \frac{23}{33}$$

In this problem, you cannot subtract 11/33 from 1/33, so you must borrow 1 or 33/33 from 100, add it to 1/33 = 34/33.
Next, subtract as in the other problems.

d.
$$175\frac{4}{6} = 175\frac{4}{6}$$
$$148\frac{1}{3} = 148\frac{2}{6}$$
$$27\frac{2}{6} = \frac{1}{3} = 27\frac{1}{3}$$

5. *Subtract the following decimal fractions.*

   a.   950.00
      − 250.25

       699.75

Line up the decimal points and numbers in straight lines and then proceed as with whole numbers.

Remember to bring the decimal point down.

   b.   0.050
      −0.025

      0.025

A zero to the left of the decimal indicates there is no whole number. The number is less than 1.

   c.   16.230
      −14.293

       1.937

   d.   2.80
      −0.95

       1.85

6. *Multiply the following fractions.*

   a. $\dfrac{2}{4} \times \dfrac{4}{6} = \dfrac{8}{24} = \dfrac{1}{3}$

(1) Multiply the numerators and denominators. It is not necessary to find a common denominator. (2) When multiplying or dividing fractions, reduce the fractions to the lowest term.

   b. $\dfrac{1}{2} \times \dfrac{1}{3} = \dfrac{1}{6}$

   c. $5\dfrac{1}{6} \times \dfrac{1}{8} =$

      $\dfrac{31}{6} \times \dfrac{1}{8} = \dfrac{31}{48}$

Mixed numbers, i.e. 5 1/6, must be changed to an improper fraction. Multiply the whole number by the denominator and add to the numerator. Multiply the numerators and the denominators.

   d. $4\dfrac{4}{5} \times 2\dfrac{1}{5} \times 8\dfrac{1}{4} = \dfrac{24}{5} \times \dfrac{11}{5} \times \dfrac{33}{4} = \dfrac{8712}{100} = 87\dfrac{12}{100} = 87\dfrac{3}{25}$

7. *Multiply the following decimals.*

   a.   1.5 multiplicand
      $\times$ 3 multiplier

      4.5 product

Multiply decimal fractions as you would multiply whole numbers. To determine where to place the decimal point in the product, count the number of places to the right of the decimal in both the multiplicand and the multiplier. The number of decimal places in the product is equal to the sum of the decimal places in the multiplicand and the multiplier.

b.
$$\begin{array}{r} 0.05 \\ \times\ 1.5 \\ \hline 25 \\ 5\ \ \\ \hline 0.075 \end{array}$$

c.
$$\begin{array}{r} 36.284 \\ \times\ 7.21 \\ \hline 36284 \\ 72568\ \ \\ 253988\ \ \ \ \\ \hline 261.60764 \end{array}$$

d.
$$\begin{array}{r} 0.0033 \\ 6.02 \\ \hline 66 \\ 0\ \ \\ 198\ \ \ \ \\ \hline 0.019866 \end{array}$$

8. *Divide the following fractions.*

Dividend Divisor

a. $\dfrac{1}{2} \div \dfrac{1}{3} = \dfrac{1}{2} \times \dfrac{3}{1} = \dfrac{3}{2} = 1\dfrac{1}{2}$

To divide fractions, invert the divisor (the number by which you are dividing) and then proceed as in multiplication.

b. $\dfrac{1}{150} \div \dfrac{1}{2} =$

$\dfrac{1}{150} \times \dfrac{2}{1} = \dfrac{1}{75}$

c. $3\dfrac{3}{4} \div \dfrac{2}{3} =$

$\dfrac{15}{4} \times \dfrac{3}{2} = \dfrac{45}{8} = 5\dfrac{5}{8}$

Change the mixed number to an improper fraction and divide by inverting the divisor.

d. $\dfrac{1\frac{1}{2}}{\frac{7}{8}} \div \dfrac{1\frac{1}{3}}{2\frac{1}{2}} =$

Change the mixed numbers to improper fractions. Work the problem as if it contained whole numbers. Divide by inverting the 4/3 over 5/2 and multiply the fractions.

$\dfrac{\frac{3}{2}}{\frac{7}{8}} \div \dfrac{\frac{4}{3}}{\frac{5}{2}} =$

$\dfrac{\frac{3}{2}}{\frac{7}{8}} \times \dfrac{\frac{5}{2}}{\frac{4}{3}} = \dfrac{\frac{15}{4}}{\frac{28}{24}} = \dfrac{15}{\cancel{4}_{1}} \times \dfrac{\cancel{24}^{6}}{28} = \dfrac{90}{28} = 3\dfrac{3}{14}$

9. *Divide the following decimals.*

               Divisor   25.8   Quotient

a. $64.5 \div 2.5 =$

$$2.5 \overline{)64.5\,0} \quad \text{Dividend}$$

$$\begin{array}{r} 25.8 \\ 2.5 \overline{)64.5\,0} \\ \underline{50} \\ 145 \\ \underline{125} \\ 200 \\ \underline{200} \end{array}$$

To divide decimal fractions, first clear the decimal places from the divisor, making it a whole number (i.e., move the decimal 1 place to the right). Next, use a caret mark (∧) to indicate the new position of the decimal point; because you have moved the decimal point in the divisor to the right, you must move the decimal point in the dividend an equal number of places to the right. Place the decimal point in the answer (quotient) directly above the decimal point in the dividend.

b. $2.5 \div 0.01 =$

$$\begin{array}{r} 250 \\ 0.01 \overline{)2.50} \end{array}$$

c. $12.075 \div 2.5 =$

$$\begin{array}{r} 4.83 \\ 2.5 \overline{)12.075} \\ \underline{100} \\ 207 \\ \underline{200} \\ 75 \\ \underline{75} \end{array}$$

d. $0.065 \div 10 =$

$$\begin{array}{r} 0.0065 \\ 10 \overline{)0.0650} \end{array}$$

10. *Solve for N using a formula.*

a. $\dfrac{24}{48} \times 5 = N$

Multiply the fraction in the usual manner to solve for N.

$$\overset{3}{\underset{6}{\cancel{\dfrac{24}{48}}}} \times \dfrac{5}{1} = \dfrac{15}{6} = 2\dfrac{1}{2}$$

b. $\dfrac{120}{60} \times 2.2 = N$

$$\overset{2}{\underset{1}{\cancel{\dfrac{120}{60}}}} \times \dfrac{2.2}{1} = 4.4$$

c. $\dfrac{3.5}{1.75} \times 5 = N$

$$\dfrac{3.5}{1.75} \times \dfrac{5}{1} = \dfrac{17.5}{1.75} = 10$$

$$\begin{array}{r} 10 \\ 1.75. \overline{\smash{\big)}\,17.50.} \\ \underline{175} \\ 00 \end{array}$$

d. $\dfrac{32}{16} \times N = 60$

$$\dfrac{\overset{2}{\cancel{32}}}{\underset{1}{\cancel{16}}} \times N = 60$$

$$\dfrac{2}{1} \div \dfrac{2}{1} \times N = 60 \div \dfrac{2}{1}$$

$$\dfrac{2}{1} \times \dfrac{1}{2} \times N = \overset{30}{\cancel{60}} \times \dfrac{1}{\underset{1}{\cancel{2}}} = 30$$

$$N = 30$$

In this problem, the unknown factor is multiplied by the fraction. To find the value of N, divide both sides of the equation by 32/16 (or 2/1 if you prefer to reduce the fraction 32/16 = 2/1). To check the equation, substitute 30 for N; multiply to see if the answer is 60.

11. *Solve for X using ratio and proportion.*

a. A *proportion* consists of two ratios that have equivalent value. A *ratio* consists of two numbers separated by a colon, indicating a relationship exists between the two numbers.

$$5 : 20 :: 2 : X$$

means

extremes

$$5\,X = 40$$
$$\dfrac{5}{5}\,X = \dfrac{40}{5}$$
$$X = 8$$

or

$$\dfrac{5}{20} \times \dfrac{2}{X}$$

$$5X = 40$$
$$\dfrac{5X}{5} = \dfrac{40}{5}$$
$$X = 8$$

To solve this sort of problem, multiply the extremes (the two outside numbers) and then multiply the means (the two inside numbers). Solve for X. In a true proportion, the product of the means equals the product of the extremes. You may check your answer by substituting the value of X into the proportion and multiply the means and then multiply the extremes. They should be equal. The two ratios in the proportion may be set up as fractions. Cross multiply. In order to be consistent, keep the unknown factor on the left side and the known factor on the right side of the equation.

b. $\dfrac{1}{6} : 1 :: X : 1\dfrac{1}{2}$

$1X = \dfrac{1}{6} \times \dfrac{3}{2}$

$1X = \dfrac{3}{12}$

$X = \dfrac{1}{4}$

or

$\dfrac{\frac{1}{6}}{1} = \dfrac{X}{1\frac{1}{2}}$

$\dfrac{\frac{1}{6}}{1} = \dfrac{X}{\frac{3}{2}}$

$1X = \dfrac{3}{12} = \dfrac{1}{4}$

c. $\dfrac{2.5}{X} :: \dfrac{5}{10}$ or 2.5 : X :: 5 : 10

$5X = 25$

$X = 5$

d. $\dfrac{X}{\frac{3}{4}} = \dfrac{\frac{7}{9}}{\frac{21}{24}}$

$\dfrac{21}{24}X = \dfrac{21}{36}$

$\dfrac{21}{24} \div \dfrac{21}{24} X = \dfrac{21}{36} \div \dfrac{21}{24}$

$\dfrac{\cancel{21}}{\cancel{24}} \times \dfrac{\cancel{24}}{\cancel{21}} X = \dfrac{\cancel{21}^{1}}{\cancel{36}_{9}} \times \dfrac{\cancel{24}^{6}}{\cancel{21}_{1}}$

$X = \dfrac{6}{9} = \dfrac{2}{3}$

or

$X : \dfrac{3}{4} :: \dfrac{7}{9} : \dfrac{21}{24}$

12. *Write the following Arabic numbers as Roman numerals.*

		Review
a. 8	VIII	I = 1
b. 3	III	V = 5
c. 21	XXI	X = 10
d. 50	L	L = 50
		C = 100
		M = 1,000

13. *Write the following Roman numerals as Arabic numbers.*
   a. CIV   104
   b. XL   40
   c. MCMLXXXI   1,981
   d. XV   15

14. *Change the following units to the indicated equivalents.*

	Percentage	Decimal	Fraction	Ratio
a.	10%	*0.10	*1/10	*1:10
b.	*65%	0.65	*13/20	*13:20
c.	*25%	*0.25	1/4	*1:4
d.	*0.2%	*0.002	*1/500	.01:500

   a. To change a percentage value to a decimal value, move the decimal point two places to the left and drop the percent sign.
   10% = 0.10
   0.1 is read one tenth, or the fraction 1/10. The ratio is formed from the fraction 1/10.

   b. The percent is determined from the decimal by moving the decimal point two places to the right and adding a percent sign. The fraction is determined by placing the decimal over 100, 65/100, and reducing the fraction, 65/100 = 13/20.

*Answers to Question 14 on p. xv.

c. The decimal is determined from the fraction by dividing the numerator by the denominator.

$$\frac{1}{4} = 4\overline{)1.00} \quad \begin{array}{r} .25 \\ \hline \end{array}$$

$$\begin{array}{r} \underline{8} \\ 20 \end{array}$$

d. The fraction is determined from the ratio by writing the ratio as a fraction. 1:500 becomes $\dfrac{1}{500}$

If you have mastered all of the problems in this self evaluation test, you are ready to learn how to calculate dosage and solutions problems. If you fail to understand how to solve any group of problems, seek help from someone who understands the techniques, or refer to a basic arithmetic book. You *must* master the arithmetic, for this is basic to accurate dosage calculation.

INTRODUCTION TO PHARMACOLOGY

In 1975 Congress passed the Metric Conversion Act which states that the United States will convert to the metric system of weights and measures at some indefinite time in the future. We see some evidence of conversion to the metric system where bottling companies are supplying soft drinks in metric measures; gasoline is being sold by the liter; highway mileage signs are being posted in kilometers. In addition, modern measuring cups are inscribed with both metric and household measures.

In medicine, too, the trend has been toward the metric system. All drugs are now manufactured in metric units. Some drugs that have been used for many years also carry the apothecaries' equivalent on the label. Physicians trained in apothecaries' units still order drugs by this system of measurement. Therefore, nurses must know both the metric and the apothecaries' systems to safely administer medications. In a recent survey of the hospitals and nursing homes in the state of Maryland, and in some other states as well, I found that the apothecaries' system is still being used by many physicians in ordering drugs.

In addition to these two systems, the nurse must be familiar with the household system used for self-medication in the home. Each of these three systems has different symbols and abbreviations. *The three systems are only approximate equivalents; they are not equal.* Each of these systems of measurement will be discussed separately in the following chapters.

[Handwritten notes at top:]

gram - weight
Meter - length
Liter - volume

Main 3 units in Metric System

Base or units 4 multiples 100ths
deka - 10
hecto - 100
Kilo 1000

Basic / fraction
gram / deci 0.1
meter / centi 0.01
Liter / milli 0.0001
micro 0.0001
less than

1   The Metric System

[handwritten: Multip of 10]

OBJECTIVES

After studying the content of this chapter, the student will be able to:

1. *Name the basic units of the metric system used in nursing.*
2. *Interpret the abbreviations for metric units.*
3. *Write the units of weight and measure using the metric system abbreviations.*
4. *Convert larger metric units to smaller metric units.*
5. *Convert smaller metric units to larger metric units.*

The metric system is a uniform system of weights and measures based on multiples of 10. Because of the ease of working within a decimal system, the metric system is used for most scientific and medical measurements.

The basic units of measure in the metric system are: the *gram* (Gm, gm or g), a unit of weight used for measuring solids; the *liter* (L or l), a unit of volume used for measuring liquids; the *meter* (M or m), a unit of linear measure used to measure length or distance.

Multiples of the basic units are designated by the prefixes deka- (10), hecto- (100) and kilo- (1000).

Fractions of the units are designated by the prefixes deci- (0.1), centi- (0.01), milli- (0.001), and micro- (0.000001).

The four metric weights frequently used by nurses are stated from the largest to the smallest weight: the kilogram (kg); gram (g or gm); the milligram (mg or mgm); and the microgram (mcg or μg).

There are only two units of volume used by nurses. They are the liter (L) or the milliliter (ml).

The units of length used by nurses are the centimeter and the millimeter.

METRIC CONVERSIONS

Weight	Liquid Volume	Length
Kilogram = Kg or kg	Liter = L or l	Centimeter = cm
Gram = Gm or g or gm	*Cubic centimeter = cc	Millimeter = mm
Milligram = mg or mgm	*Milliliter = ml	
Microgram = mcg or μg		

---

*The cubic centimeter and the milliliter are considered equivalent and are used interchangeably, 1 ml = 1 cc.

SYSTEM	MULTIPLES OF THE UNIT			UNIT		FRACTIONS OF THE UNIT					
	THOUSANDS	HUNDREDS	TENS	UNIT	DECIMAL POINT	TENTHS	HUNDREDTHS	THOUSANDTHS	TEN THOUSANDTHS	HUNDRED THOUSANDTHS	MILLIONTHS
DECIMAL	0	0	0	0	.	0	0	0	0	0	0
METRIC	*KILO	HECTO	DEKA	*METERS, LITERS, OR GRAMS		DECI	CENTi	*MILLI			*MICRO

Equivalents. Each of these units differs from the next by 1000.

1000 gm = 1 kg (100 gm in each 0.1 kg)   1000 gram
1000 mg = 1 gm (100 mg in each 0.1 gm)   0.001 gram
1000 mcg = 1 mg (100 mcg in each 0.1 mg)   0.001 milligram or 0.000001 gram

Conversion Within the Metric System. To change from a larger unit to a smaller unit:

kg to gm
L to ml   *multiply by 1,000*
gm to mg
mg to mcg

> This is the same as moving the decimal point 3 places to the right.

To change from a smaller unit to a larger unit:

gm to kg
ml to L   *divide by 1000*
mg to gm
mcg to mg

> This is the same as moving the decimal point 3 places to the left.

hehe/p

Symbols that may help you to remember:

larger ⟶ smaller   to go from the larger measure to the smaller measure, move the decimal point the way the arrow points 3 places to the right.

smaller ⟵ larger   to go from the smaller measure to the larger one, move the decimal point the way the arrow points 3 places to the left.

The wide end of the arrow represents the larger measure. The small end or point of the arrow represents the smaller measure and points in the direction the decimal point is to be moved.

get help

EXAMPLES

1. Convert liters to milliliters

    4 L = 4000 ml
      Multiply 4 by 1000 = 4000 ml *OR*
      Move the decimal point 3 places to the right 4.000 = 4000 ml

                A liter is larger L ⟶ ml is smaller

2. Convert milliliters to liters

    3000 ml = 3 L
      Divide 3000 ml by 1000
$$\frac{3\ L}{1000\ )\overline{3000\ ml}}\quad OR$$
      Move the decimal point 3 places to the left   3000. ml = 3 L

            Milliliters are smaller ⟵ Liters are larger than ml

3. Convert grams to milligrams

    20 grams × 1000 = 20,000 mg
      Move the decimal point 3 places to the right
      20 gm   20.000 mg.
      larger measure ⟶ smaller measure

4. Convert milligrams to grams

    250 mg ÷ 1000 = 0.25 gm *OR*
      Move the decimal point 3 places to the left   250 mg = 0.25 gm

                          ⟵

5. Convert milligrams to micrograms

    0.04 mg × 1000 = 40 micrograms
    Move decimal point 3 places to the right   0.040 mg = 40 mcg

6. Convert micrograms to milligrams

    25 mcg ÷ 1000 = 25   25 mg = 0.025 mg

    Move the decimal point 3 places to the left

PROBLEMS: METRIC SYSTEM CONVERSION

Always place a zero in front of your decimal point when there is no whole number there. The zero gives emphasis to the decimal and helps prevent dosage errors.

1. Liters to milliliters
    a. 1 L   = _1.000 ML_
    b. 0.5 L = _5000 M_
    c. 4.5 L = _4500 Ml_
    d. 0.125 L= _125 mL_
    e. 3.25 L = _325 ml_

2. Milliliters to liters
    a. 500 ml = _.05 L_
    b. 60 ml   = _0.06 L_
    c. 5 ml   = _0.005 L_
    d. 1300 ml = _1.3 L_
    e. 4225 ml = _4.225 L_

3. Grams to milligrams
    a. 2500 gm = _2,500,000 mg_
    b. 0.5 gm = _5000 MG_
    c. 1.2 gm = _____
    d. 0.065 gm = _65 mg_
    e. 50 gm   = _____

4. Milligrams to grams
    a. 1.5 mg = _0.0015 gR_
    b. 3 mg   = _____
    c. 0.5 mg = _____
    d. 400 mg = _____
    e. 6000 mg = _____

5. Kilograms to grams
    a. 5 kg   = _5000 gR_
    b. 30 kg = _30,000 gL_
    c. 400 kg = _400,00 gR_
    d. 3.5 kg = _gR_
    e. 0.4 kg = _4000 gL_

6. Grams to kilograms
    a. 50 gm   = _0.05 kil_
    b. 25 gm   = _0.025 kil_
    c. 2.2 gm = _0.0022_
    d. 2500 gm = _2.5_
    e. 425 gm = _0.425_

7. Milligrams to micrograms
    a. 0.6 mg   = _600 mcg_
    b. 0.420 mg = _420 mcg_
    c. 250 mg   = _250,000 mcg_
    d. 125 mg   = _125,000 mcg_
    e. 0.015 mg = _1515 mcg_

8. Micrograms to milligrams
    a. 6 mcg   = _0.006 mg_
    b. 43 mcg   = _0.043 mg_
    c. 225 mcg   = _0.225 mg_
    d. 4513 mcg = _4.513 mg_
    e. 20,280 mcg = _20.58 mg_

Quiz on Metric System & trade & generic
definition allergy & uses

ANSWERS: METRIC SYSTEM CONVERSION

1. Liters to milliliters

    a. 1 L   = 1000 ml
    b. 0.5 L   = 500 ml
    c. 4.5 L   = 4500 ml
    d. 0.125 L = 125 ml
    e. 3.25 L   = 3250 ml

2. Milliliters to liters

    a. 500 ml   = 0.5 L
    b. 60 ml   = 0.06 L
    c. 5 ml   = 0.005 L
    d. 1300 ml = 1.3 L
    e. 4225 ml = 4.225 L

3. Grams to milligrams

    a. 2500 gm   = 2,500,000 mg
    b. 0.5 gm   = 500 mg
    c. 1.2 gm   = 1200 mg
    d. 0.065 gm = 65 mg
    e. 50 gm   = 50,000 mg

4. Milligrams to grams

    a. 1.5 mg   = 0.0015 gm
    b. 3 mg   = 0.003 gm
    c. 0.5 mg   = 0.0005 gm
    d. 400 mg   = 0.4 gm
    e. 6000 mg = 6 gm

5. Kilograms to grams

    a. 5 kg   = 5000 gm
    b. 30 kg   = 30,000 gm
    c. 400 kg   = 400,000 gm
    d. 3.5 kg   = 3500 gm
    e. 0.4 kg   = 400 gm

6. Grams to kilograms

    a. 50 gm   = 0.05 kg
    b. 25 gm   = 0.025 kg
    c. 2.2 gm   = 0.0022 kg
    d. 2500 gm = 2.5 kg
    e. 425 gm   = 0.425 kg

7. Milligrams to micrograms

    a. 0.6 mg   = 600 mcg
    b. 0.420 mg = 420 mcg
    c. 250 mg   = 250,000 mcg
    d. 125 mg   = 125,000 mcg
    e. 0.015 mg = 15 mcg

8. Micrograms to milligrams

    a. 6 mcg   = 0.006 mg
    b. 43 mcg   = 0.043 mg
    c. 225 mcg   = 0.225 mg
    d. 4513 mcg   = 4.513 mg
    e. 20,280 mcg = 20.28 mg

2 Apothecaries' System

OBJECTIVES

After completing this chapter, the student will be able to:

1. *Name the basic measures used in the apothecaries' system for weight and for volume*
2. *Read and interpret the abbreviations for apothecaries' symbols and numbers*
3. *Write the symbols and the correct dosage using Roman numerals*
4. *Set up and work dosage problems to obtain the correct dosage to be administered*
5. *Convert from one apothecaries' measure to another.*

The apothecaries' system of weights and measures was brought to America from England by the first colonists. The apothecary shop sold herbs and other medicines to cure the ills of humankind. This system of weights has been used by pharmacists to prepare medications throughout our history. Today, however, the metric system is fast becoming the universal system of weights and measures, and has largely replaced the apothecaries' system in the United States.

Drug and pharmaceutical companies now use the metric system of weights and measures in labeling their products. The label of drugs that were originally produced under the apothecaries' system still state the apothecaries' equivalent on the label, in addition to the metric equivalent. Examples of these older drugs are codeine, phenobarbital, atropine and aspirin, to name only a few. Many physicians, trained in the apothecaries' system of measurement, still write orders under this system. However, until all drugs are ordered in the metric system, nurses must learn both the metric and apothecaries' systems.

APOTHECARIES' SYSTEM UNITS OF VOLUME AND WEIGHT

In the apothecaries' system the basic unit of weight is the grain. Originally the grain was equal in weight to a grain of wheat. The next largest measurement is the scruple, which, since it is not used in medicine, will not be discussed here. The next larger measurement is the dram. The dram is used in both liquid and solid measurement. One dram is equal to 60 grains. There are eight drams in the next larger measure, which is the ounce. The pint, the quart, and the gallon are the next larger measures, listed here in the order of increasing size. There are 12 ounces in an apothecaries' pound in contrast with the avoirdupois pound familiar to most people which contains 16 ounces.

The basic unit for volume is the minim. The minim is approximately equal to the amount of water that would weigh 1 grain. Since a minim is approximately equivalent in weight to the grain, they are considered equal. The fluid dram, the fluid ounce, the pint, the quart, and the gallon are the units of volume listed in order of increasing size.

The symbol for minim is ℩

The symbol for grain is gr

The symbol for dram is ʒ (The dram is smaller than the ounce—the symbol is smaller)

The symbol for ounce is ℥ (The ounce is larger than the dram—the symbol is larger)

O is the symbol for pint and comes from the Latin octarius meaning 1/8 of a gallon

C comes from the Latin word conguis meaning the container for 1 gallon.

When apothecaries' symbols are used, the amount is expressed in Roman numerals. The Roman numeral may be written in lower case numerals. They are written after the apothecaries' symbol.

ʒ iv	= 4 drams
℩ iii	= 3 minims
gr v	= 5 grains
℥ xxx	= 30 ounces
O i	= 1 pint

Fractions are expressed in Arabic numerals after the symbol—gr 1/8. The symbol ss comes from the Latin word semis, meaning one half—gr ss = gr 1/2; gr viiss = gr 7 1/2. You may see a line over the Roman numerals—gr $\overline{\text{xiiss}}$ = 12 1/2 grains. Dots are placed above the bar to distinguish the lowercase i's from small "el"s, meaning 50.

If Arabic numbers are used in place of Roman numerals the Arabic number is written in front of the apothecaries' unit 6 1/2 grains. The only exception to this rule is a fraction, which is written after the apothecaries' symbol—gr 1/4; gr 1/8.

APOTHECARIES' EQUIVALENT TABLE

Units of Volume

60 minims ℩lx	= 1 fluid dram f ʒ i
8 fluid drams f ʒ viii	= 1 ounce f ℥ i
16 fluid ounces f ℥ xvi	= 1 pint pt or O i
2 pints O ii	= 1 quart qt i
32 fluid ounces f ℥ xxxii	= 1 quart qt i
4 quarts	= 1 gallon gal or C i

Units of Weight

60 grains	gr lx	=	1 dram	ℨi
8 drams	ℨviii	=	1 ounce	℥i
12 ounces	℥xii	=	1 pound	

To measure liquids in the apothecaries' system use a minim glass or a medicine glass using the apothecaries' measurements. If you do not have a minim glass to measure small amounts of drugs, a minim/cc syringe may be used to measure the amount accurately.

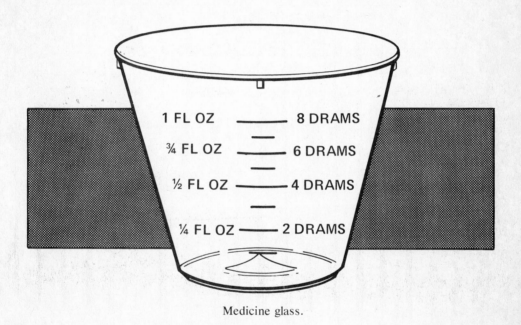

Medicine glass.

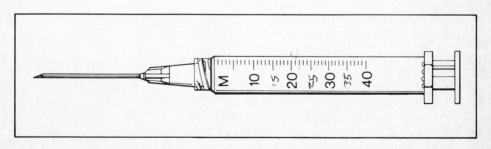

Syringe.

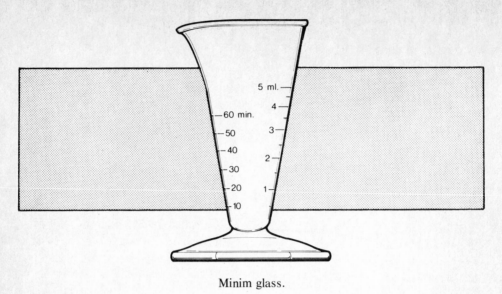

Minim glass.

PROBLEMS: APOTHECARIES' SYSTEM

1. *Read the following for practice.*

ɱ xviiss _____   f ʒ iv _____
ʒ vii _____   gr ss _____
ʒ xv _____   f ʒ ix _____
gr i _____   gr 1/300 __1/300 gr__

2. *Write the following in apothecaries' notations.*

Eleven ounces _ʒ xi_   One half fluid ounce _F ʒ ss_
4½ drams _ʒ ivss_   2 fluid drams _a f ʒ_
1 pint _O i_   One-hundred-forty minims _ɱ xl_
7 gallons _C i_   Two quarts _____

3. *Equivalents.*

1 qt   = _____ pt   ʒ iv   = _____ gr
ɱ xxx   = _____ f dram   ʒ iss   = _____ ʒ
gr lx   = _____ ʒ   C i   = _____ O
ʒ viii   = _____ ʒ   O iv   = _____ qt
f ʒ xvi = _____ O   pt iii   = _____ f ʒ
ɱ xc   = _____ f ʒ   f ʒ ii   = _____ f ʒ
ʒ ii   = _____ gr   gr xxx = _____ ʒ
f ʒ ivss = _____ f ʒ   lb iss   = _____ ʒ (troy)
1/2 gal = _____ qt   120 gr   = _____ drams
O X   = _____ gal   pt iiss = _____ ʒ

ANSWERS: APOTHECARIES' SYSTEM

1. *Read the following for practice.*

ℳ xviiss	17½ minims	f ℨ iv	4 fluid drams
ℨ vii	7 drams	gr ss	½ grain
℥ xv	15 ounces	f ℥ ix	9 fluid ounces
gr i	1 grain	gr 1/300	1/300 grain

2. *Write the following in apothecaries' notations.*

Eleven ounces	℥ xi	One half fluid ounce	f ℥ ss
4½ drams	ℨ ivss	2 fluid drams	f ℨ ii
1 pint	1 pt or O i	One-hundred-forty minims	ℳ cxl
7 gallons	C vii	Two quarts	2 qts.

3. *Equivalents.*

1 qt	=	2	pt	℥ iv	=	240	gr
ℳ xxx	=	½	f dram	℥ iss	=	12	ℨ
gr lx	=	1	ℨ	C i	=	8	O
ℨ viii	=	1	℥	O iv	=	2	qt
f ℥ xvi	=	1	O	pt iii	=	48	f ℥
ℳ xc	=	1½	f ℨ	f ℥ ii	=	16	f ℨ
ℨ ii	=	120	gr	gr xxx	=	½	ℨ
f ℥ ivss	=	36	f ℨ	lb iss	=	18	℥ (troy)
1/2 gal	=	2	qt	120 gr	=	2	drams
O X	=	1¼	gal	pt iiss	=	40	℥

In Apothecaries System

$\frac{D}{H} \times V$

Pherobar
gr $\frac{1}{55} = \frac{1}{2}$ or phen —
gr $\frac{1}{4}$

$\dfrac{\frac{1}{2}}{\frac{1}{4}} \times 1 = 2$ or $\frac{1}{2} + \frac{\frac{2}{4}}{1} = 2$

gr $\frac{1}{600}$
gr $\frac{1}{300}$ $V = V$ $\dfrac{\frac{1}{600}}{2} \atop \dfrac{\frac{1}{300}}{1} = 1 = \frac{1}{2}$

$\begin{array}{c}15\\900\\3\,800\end{array}$

gr $\frac{1}{150}$ $\dfrac{\frac{1}{150}}{\frac{1}{300}} \times 1$ 2 Tabs

gr $\frac{1}{300}$ $\frac{1}{300}$
      2

gr $\frac{1}{4}$

gr $\frac{1}{2}$

3 Household System

OBJECTIVES

After completing this unit, the student will be able to:

1. Name the basic units of measure in the household system.
2. Read and interpret the abbreviations for household symbols and numbers.
3. Write dosages using household symbols.
4. Convert from one household measure to another.
5. Work dosage problems within the household system.

The household system is used for administering medication in the home. It is also used in determining patient oral intake from the food tray or water pitcher. The intake is then converted to the metric equivalent. This system is not a complete system because it contains only units of volume. The units are the glass, cup, tablespoon, teaspoon, and drop. There is a lack of standardization in the size of these utensils, so the size may vary considerably.

A drop varies in size depending on the temperature of the liquid, the viscosity of the liquid, the angle at which the dropper is held, and the diameter of the bore of the dropper. Drops and minims are thought to be equivalent, but because of the variations in drop sizes they should never be used interchangeably.

The teaspoon varies in size from 4 to 5 ml or more. The American Standards Institute sets the standard for an American teaspoon at 5 ml. For household measurements, 3 teaspoons equal 1 tablespoon. A true calibrated tablespoon equals 4 teaspoons.

If a medication is to be measured by the household system, the physician must order the drug in household measures. If the patient's condition, the potency of the drug, or other factors require greater accuracy of measurement, the nurse may help the patient to secure the appropriate calibrated measuring equipment.

ACCEPTED STANDARDS

60 drops (gtt) = 1 teaspoonful (t) or tsp
3 teaspoonfuls = 1 tablespoonful (T) or Tbs
2 tablespoonfuls = 1 ounce or oz

6 fluid ounces = 1 teacupful
8 fluid ounces = 1 glassful
16 ounces = 1 pound

Pints and quarts are found in the home but these are considered apothecaries' measures.

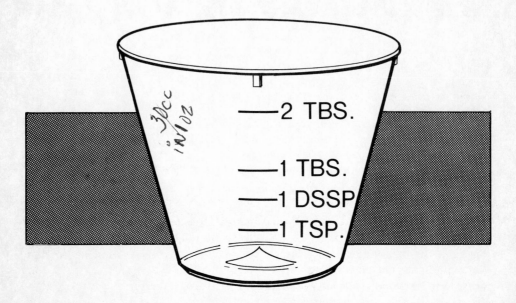

PROBLEMS: EQUIVALENTS

6 t	= _____ T	12 oz	= _____ glasses
18 t	= _____ oz	4 T	= _____ oz
4 oz	= _____ T	1 glass	= _____ oz
12 oz	= _____ cups	3 cups	= _____ oz

ANSWERS: EQUIVALENTS

6 t	= 2 T	12 oz	= 1½ glasses
18 t	= 3 oz	4 T	= 2 oz
4 oz	= 8 T	1 glass	= 8 oz
12 oz	= 2 cups	3 cups	= 18 oz

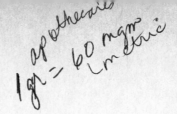
apothecaries
1 gr = 60 mgm
in metric

4   Conversion Between the Apothecaries' and the Metric System

OBJECTIVES

After completing this chapter, the student will be able to:

1. *State the ratio for conversion between grains and grams.*
2. *Work problems to convert grains to grams.*
3. *Work problems to convert grams to grains.*
4. *State the ratio for conversion between milligrams and grains.*
5. *Work problems to convert milligrams to grains.*
6. *Work problems to convert grains to milligrams.*
7. *Explain the inequivalence of the apothecaries' and metric systems.*

Medications that have been in use for many years list both the metric and apothecaries' equivalents on the label. Examples are ferrous sulfate, phenobarbital, nitroglycerin, and codeine to name only a few. The two systems are only approximately equivalent, so you will see discrepancies on the labels. One grain in the apothecaries' system is equal to 0.0648 grams. The accepted approximate metric equivalent is 60*, 64, or 65 milligrams depending on how the number is rounded off. For example, sometimes you will have an order for 300 mg of ferrous sulfate and the preparation stocked is marked 325 mg. Both 300 mg and 325 mg equal 5 grains. Request that the physician write the order according to the strength supplied in the hospital. If the order is written as 5 grains, either strength (above) is correct.

$$60 \text{ mg} \times 5 \text{ gr} = 300 \text{ mg}$$
$$64 \text{ mg} \times 5 \text{ gr} = 320 \text{ mg}$$
$$65 \text{ mg} \times 5 \text{ gr} = 325 \text{ mg}$$

To convert from milligrams to grains or grains to milligrams, use the ratio 1 gr : 60 mg.

Convert 5 gr to milligrams
60 mg : 1 gr : : X mg : 5 gr
1X = 300 mg

Convert 300 mg to grains
60 mg : 1gr : : 300 mg : X gr
$$60X = 300$$
$$\frac{60}{60} X = \frac{300}{60}$$
$$X = 5 \text{ gr}$$

*For conversion purposes in this book, use 60 mg = 1 grain as the basic ratio.

To convert from grams to grains, or grains to grams, use the ratio 15 gr:1 gm. Remember that conversions from one system to another are only approximate equivalents.

Convert 60 gr to grams
$$15 \text{ gr} : 1 \text{ gm} : : 60 \text{ gr} : X \text{gm}$$
$$15X = 60$$
$$\frac{15}{15}X = \frac{60}{15}$$
$$X = 4 \text{ gm}$$

Convert 4 gm to grains
$$15 \text{ gr} : 1 \text{ gm} : : X \text{ gr} : 4 \text{ gm}$$
$$X = 60 \text{ gr}$$

EQUIVALENTS

Apothecaries' System	Metric Equivalent	Approximate Metric Equivalents Used By Nurses
1 grain	0.0648 mg	60 or 64 or 65 mg
15.432 gr	1 gram	1 gram
1 minim	0.06161 ml	0.06 ml
60 minims	3.697 ml	4 ml
1 dram	3.697 ml	4 ml
8 drams	29.5729 ml	30 ml
16 ounces = 1 pint	473.167 ml	500 ml or ½ liter
2 pints = 1 quart	946.333 ml	1000 ml or 1 liter

Examples of drugs labeled with different milligram-grain equivalences. These differences point out the fact that the apothecaries' and metric systems are not equal but are approximate equivalents. Be very careful when giving drugs ordered in one system and supplied in another system of measurement. Small differences in some drugs may produce harmful effects.

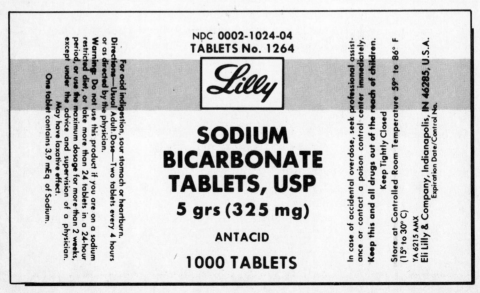

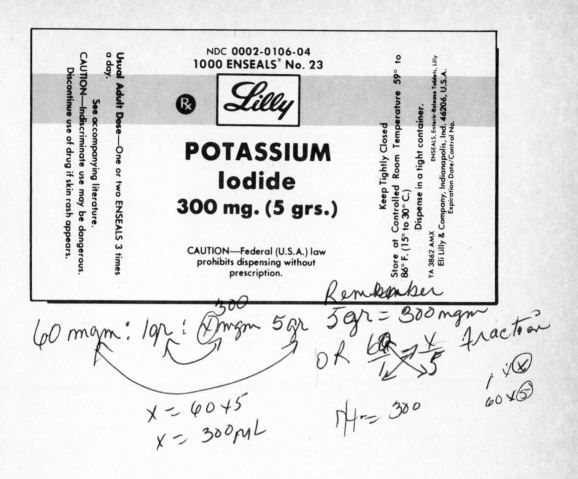

NDC 0002-0106-04
1000 ENSEALS® No. 23

℞ *Lilly*

POTASSIUM
Iodide
300 mg. (5 grs.)

CAUTION—Federal (U.S.A.) law
prohibits dispensing without
prescription.

Usual Adult Dose—One or two ENSEALS 3 times
a day.
CAUTION—Indiscriminate use may be dangerous.
Discontinue use of drug if skin rash appears.
See accompanying literature.

Keep Tightly Closed
Store at Controlled Room Temperature 59° to
86° F. (15° to 30° C.).
Dispense in a tight container.

ENSEALS, Enteric-Release Tablets, Lilly
Eli Lilly & Company, Indianapolis, Ind. 46206, U.S.A.
Expiration Date/Control No.
YA 3862 AMX

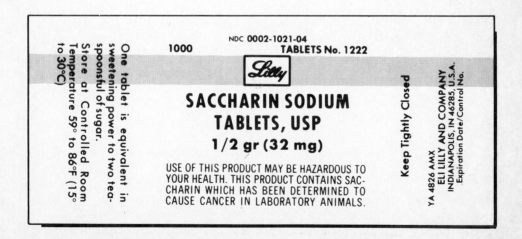

$60 \text{ mgm} : 1 \text{ gr} : X \text{ mgm} \quad 5 \text{ gr}$

Remember
$5 \text{ gr} = 300 \text{ mgm}$

or $\dfrac{60}{1} \nearrow \dfrac{X}{5}$ fraction

$\dfrac{1 \times X}{60 \times 5}$

$X = 60 \times 5$
$X = 300 \, ML$

$X = 300$

NDC 0002-1021-04
1000   **TABLETS No. 1222**

Lilly

SACCHARIN SODIUM
TABLETS, USP
1/2 gr (32 mg)

USE OF THIS PRODUCT MAY BE HAZARDOUS TO
YOUR HEALTH. THIS PRODUCT CONTAINS SAC-
CHARIN WHICH HAS BEEN DETERMINED TO
CAUSE CANCER IN LABORATORY ANIMALS.

One tablet is equivalent in
sweetening power to two tea-
spoonsful of sugar.
Store at Controlled Room
Temperature 59° to 86°F (15°
to 30°C)

Keep Tightly Closed

ELI LILLY AND COMPANY
INDIANAPOLIS, IN 46285, U.S.A.
Expiration Date/Control No.
YA 4826 AMX

NDC 0002-1032-04
1000 TABLETS No. 1545
Lilly C IV
PHENOBARBITAL TABLETS, USP
30 mg (1/2 gr)
WARNING—May be habit forming.

CAUTION—Federal (U.S.A) law prohibits dispensing without prescription.

Usual Adult Sedative Dose—15 to 30 mg 2 to 4 times a day.
Usual Adult Hypnotic Dose—100 to 200 mg

Keep Tightly Closed
Store at Controlled Room Temperature 59° to 86° F (15° to 30° C)
Dispense in a tight container.
YA 6288 AMX
Eli Lilly & Co., Indianapolis, IN 46285, U.S.A.
Expiration Date/Control No.

COMPARISON OF THE THREE SYSTEMS OF MEASURE

METRIC		APOTHECARIES'		HOUSEHOLD[1]
Volume	Weight	Volume	Weight	Volume
0.06 ml	0.06 gm or 60 mg	1 minim ℳ i	1 grain gr i	1 drop 1 gtt
1 ml	1 gm	15 or 16 minims	15 or 16 grains	
4-5 ml	4 gm	1 fluid dram f ʒ i	1 dram ʒ i	1 tsp[2]
15-16 ml[3]	15-16 gm[3]	4 fluid drams f ʒ iv	4 drams ʒ iv	1 tbsp
30-32 ml[4]	30-32 gm[4]	1 fluid ounce f ℥ i	1 ounce ℥ i	2 tbsp
180 ml		6 ounces f ℥ vi		1 teacupful
240 ml		8 ounces f ℥ viii		1 glassful
0.5 L or 500 ml[5]		16 ounces 1 pt Oi		1 pint
1 L or 1000 ml[6]		32 ounces 1 qt		1 quart
	1 kilogram		2.2 lb avoirdupois	

[1]The household system is inaccurate and should not be used for medications unless the drug is specifically ordered in household measurement.
[2]A scant teaspoon = 4 ml.   A full teaspoon = 5 ml.
[3]One-half ounce is usually considered to be 15 ml.
[4]One ounce is usually considered to be 30 ml.
[5]Pints are not exactly equal to 500 ml but this is the accepted standard used in nursing.
[6]Quarts are not exactly equal to 1000 ml but this is the accepted standard used in nursing.

APPROXIMATE EQUIVALENTS THAT NURSES SHOULD MEMORIZE

METRIC	WEIGHT APOTHECARIES'	HOUSEHOLD
0.06 gm or 60 mg	1 grain	
1 gm	15 or 16 grains	
1 kg	2.2 lb (avoirdupois)	

	VOLUME	
0.06 ml	1 minim	
1 ml	15-16 minims	
4 ml	1 dram	1 scant teaspoon
15 ml	½ ounce	1 tablespoon
30 ml	8 drams	
30 ml	1 ounce	6 or 8 teaspoons
30 ml	1 ounce	2 tablespoons
180 ml	6 ounces	1 teacupful
240 ml	8 ounces	1 glassful
0.5 L 500 ml	1 pint	
0.5 L 500 ml	16 ounces	
1 L 1000 ml	32 ounces	
1 L 1000 ml	1 quart	
4 L 4000 ml	1 gallon	

Remember these two ratios described on pages 15 and 16.
  1 grain : 60 milligram
  15 grains: 1 gram

METRIC–APOTHECARIES' CONVERSION PROBLEMS

1. The physician orders: gr v of ferrous sulfate. You have ferrous sulfate 325 mg tablet.

2. The physician orders: phenobarb gr ¼. On hand phenobarb 16 mg tablet.

3. The physician orders: ephedrine gr ⅜. On hand ephedrine 23 mg tablet.

4. The physician orders: atropine gr 1/100. On hand atropine 0.65 mg tablet.

5. The physican orders: colchicine gr 1/100. On hand colchicine 0.6 mg tablet.

6. The physician orders: thyroid 0.03 gm. On hand thyroid gr ss tablet.

7. The physican orders: codeine gr ss. On hand codeine 15 mg tablet.

8. The physician orders: seconal 0.1 gm. On hand seconal gr iss capsule.

METRIC–APOTHECARIES' CONVERSION ANSWERS

1. The physician orders gr v of ferrous sulfate. You have ferrous sulfate 325 mg.

   1 gr : 60 mg : : 5 gr : X mg   1 gr : 65 mg : : 5 gr : X mg
   $\qquad$ X = 300 mg $\qquad$ X = 325 mg

   If you use the ratio 1 gr : 65 mg X mg = 325 mg
   Both answers are correct. You may give the 325 mg tablet.

2. The physician orders phenobarb gr ¼. On hand phenobarb 16 mg.

   1 gr : 60 mg : : gr ¼ : X mg
   $$X = \frac{60}{4}$$
   X = 15 mg

   If we had used 64 mg = 1 gr
   1 gr : 64 mg : : gr ¼ : X mg
   $$X = \frac{64}{4}$$
   X = 16 mg

   Both answers are correct.
   You may use the 16 mg tablet to equal gr ¼

3. The physician orders ephedrine gr ⅜. On hand ephedrine 23 mg.

   1 gr : 60 mg : : gr ⅜ : X mg
   $$X = \frac{180}{8}$$
   X = 22.5 = 23 mg

4. The physician orders: atropine gr 1/100. On hand atropine 0.65 mg.

$$1 \text{ gr} : 60 \text{ mg} :: \text{gr } 1/100 : X \text{ mg}$$
$$X = \frac{60}{100}$$
$$X = 0.60 \text{ mg}$$

Had you used 1 gr : 65 mg instead for converting gr 1/100 would equal 0.65 mg.

5. The physician orders: colchicine gr 1/100. On hand colchicine 0.6 mg.

$$1 \text{ gr} : 60 \text{ mg} :: \text{gr } 1/100 : X \text{ mg}$$
$$1X = \frac{60}{100}$$
$$X = 0.6 \text{ mg}$$

6. The physician orders: thyroid 0.03 gm. On hand thyroid gr ss.

$$15 \text{ gr} : 1 \text{ gm} :: X \text{ gr} : 0.03 \text{ gm}$$
$$1X = .45$$
$$X = \frac{45}{100} = \frac{9}{20} = \text{Approx. } 1/2 \text{ gr}$$
$$0.03 \text{ gm} = 30 \text{ mg}$$
$$1 \text{ gr} : 60 \text{ mg} :: X \text{ gr} : 30 \text{ mg}$$
$$60X = 30$$
$$X = 30/60 = \tfrac{1}{2} \text{ gr}.$$

7. The physician orders: codeine gr ss. On hand codeine 15 mg.

$$1 \text{ gr} : 60 \text{ mg} :: \text{gr } \tfrac{1}{2} : X \text{ mg}$$
$$1X = \frac{60}{2}$$
$$X = 30 \text{ mg}$$

Give 2 tablets   15 mg × 2 tab = 30 mg = gr ss

8. The physician orders: seconal 0.1 gm. On hand seconal 1½ gr.

$$15 \text{ gr} : 1 \text{ gm} :: X \text{ gr} : 0.1 \text{ gm}$$
$$1X = 1.5 \text{ gr}$$
$$X = 1\tfrac{1}{2} \text{ gr}$$

Ordered	$\frac{D}{H} \times V I$	On hand
1 gr 1/300		gr 1/150 Tab
2.40 mgr		40 mgr / 1 ml Tab
gr 1/6		gr 1/12 Tab
0.3 Gm		100 mgr Tab
0.5 Gm		250 mgr Tab

Quiz Report H

5   Reading Drug Bottle Labels

OBJECTIVES

After completing this chapter, the student will be able to:

1. *Identify the trade or proprietary name of a drug.*
2. *Identify the generic name.*
3. *Identify the dosage strength of the medication.*
4. *Identify the number of tablets or volume of a drug in a bottle of medication.*
5. *Identify the usual dosage of the drug.*
6. *Identify special precautions listed relevant to law or safety.*
7. *Identify from drug labels that the drug is a controlled substance.*
8. *Identify the schedule for the controlled drug.*
9. *Identify reconstitution instructions for powdered or crystalline drugs.*
10. *Identify the route of administration for the drug.*
11. *Identify storage instructions.*
12. *Identify the manufacturer's name.*
13. *Identify the expiration date.*

DRUGS

Drugs are manufactured under many different names. Nurses, physicians, and the general public may become confused by so many different names for one drug. Sometimes a brand name is so familiar and has been used for so long that nurses, physicians, and the public may think of the drug only by that name. Advertising practices make the brand names very familiar. The nurse needs to be familiar with the generic or nonproprietary name of each drug. This name never changes and may be used worldwide. It is written in lowercase letters. The proprietary or trade name is followed by a circled R, "®" indicating that the name is protected by law and may only be used by the drug manufacturing company registering the name. Sometimes TM is used after the name indicating that this is the trademark of the manufacturing company.

Pictured below are some labels illustrating some of the many different proprietary names for the drug ampicillin for oral administration. Other pharmaceutical companies have still different names.

Bristol uses the name Polycillin ®

Parke-Davis uses Amcill ®

Smith Kline & French uses SK-Ampicillin ®

Nurses must be certain they are using the correct drug. If you are in doubt about the drug, look it up in the Hospital Formulary, PDR, or nurse drug reference book. If you still cannot find the drug, call the pharmacist. He will be glad to assist you. Remember, it is better to ask questions than to make a drug error.

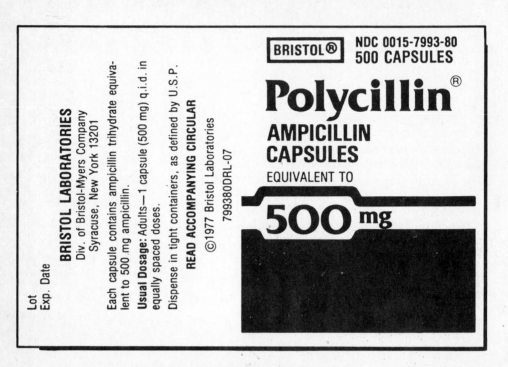

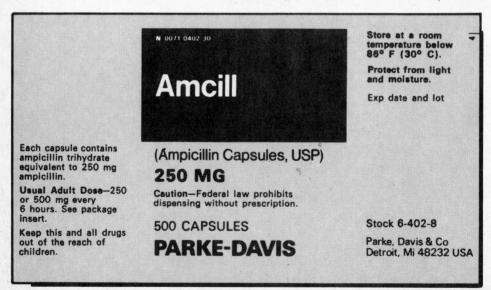

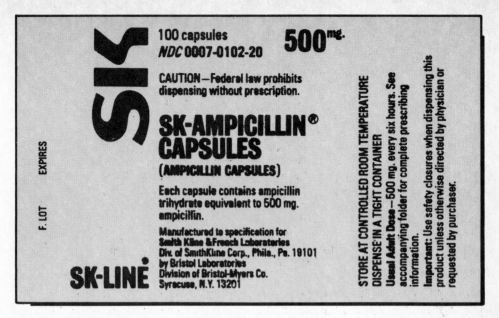

The label reads:

100 capsules
NDC 0007-0102-20
500mg.

CAUTION—Federal law prohibits dispensing without prescription.

SK-AMPICILLIN®
CAPSULES
(AMPICILLIN CAPSULES)

Each capsule contains ampicillin trihydrate equivalent to 500 mg. ampicillin.

Manufactured to specification for Smith Kline &French Laboratories Div. of SmithKline Corp., Phila., Pa. 19101 by Bristol Laboratories Division of Bristol-Myers Co. Syracuse, N.Y. 13201

SK-LINE

F. LOT   EXPIRES

STORE AT CONTROLLED ROOM TEMPERATURE DISPENSE IN A TIGHT CONTAINER

Usual Adult Dose—500 mg. every six hours. See accompanying folder for complete prescribing information.

Important: Use safety closures when dispensing this product unless otherwise directed by physician or requested by purchaser.

LABEL INFORMATION

The nurse must learn to read drug labels. The following will be found on the label.

1. Trade or brand name of the drug frequently designated with ® at the upper right of the name, indicating that the name is registered and may be used only by the manufacturer who is the legal owner of the name.

2. Under the trade name will be the generic or official name. The drug may be ordered by either name depending on the physician's preference or hospital regulation. Law requires that the generic name appear on the label.

3. On the label will be the strength of the capsule, tablet, or liquid, e.g., 25 mg capsules. This means each capsule contains 25 mg of drug.

   Drugs are usually manufactured in the strength most commonly ordered. Liquid drug labels will give the amount of drug in a given amount of solution, e.g., each ml contains 300,000 U (*drug*) or each 2.5 ml dose contains 1 gram of *drug* or 50 mg/ml which means each 1 ml of liquid contains 50 mg of the drug.

4. The number of tablets or capsules that the bottle contains will be given. (Do not confuse this with the dose.) The total amount of liquid in an ampule or a vial will be stated plus the total amount of drug in the vial or ampule, e.g., 60 milliliters or 100 capsules.

5. Usual dosage, e.g., 250 to 500 mg IV every 6 hours.

6. Special precautions are listed, e.g., Do not give to children under 3 years of age; Federal law prohibits dispensing without a prescription; Controlled Substance Schedule Number, e.g.ℂ

7. If the drug is unstable as a liquid and is dispensed as a powder or crystals, mixing instructions are given.
8. The route of administration, e.g., To be administered by intramuscular injection only.
9. Type of drug, e.g., capsule, tablet, spansule, suspension, etc.
10. Storage instructions are listed.
11. Manufacturer's name is given.
12. Expiration date.

Complete the worksheets on the following pages.

Bottle Labels

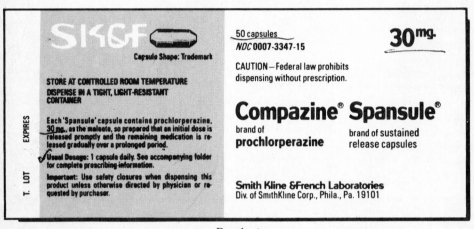

Bottle 1

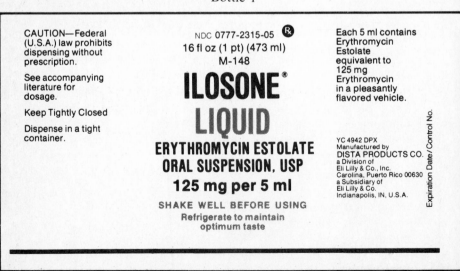

Bottle 2

Each white
and gray capsule
bears the **a** and
the Abbo-Code CI
for identification.

See package
enclosure for
dosage and full
prescribing in-
formation.

— Each capsule
contains:

clorazepate
— dipotassium
— - - - - - - 3.75 mg

U.S. Pat. No.
— Re. 28,315

100 Capsules

TRANXENE®

**3.75 Clorazepate
mg dipotassium**

Caution: Federal (U.S.A.)
law prohibits dispensing
without prescription.

a Abbott
Pharmaceuticals, Inc.
North Chicago,
IL 60064, U.S.A.

New capsule size
adopted July, 1979.

Keep bottle tightly
closed. Dispense
in a USP tight
container.

Bottle 3

USUAL DOSAGE: See accompanying circular.
Filled into container as a true
solution, then cryodesiccated.
To reconstitute, add 50 ml of 5% Dextrose Injection, or Sodium
Chloride Injection for slow intravenous injection. Discard unused
solution after 24 hours.

50 mg | No. 3330

6234806

MSD   **NDC 0006-3330-50**

**50 mg
INTRAVENOUS
SODIUM EDECRIN®**
(ETHACRYNATE SODIUM, MSD)

50 mg Ethacrynic Acid Equivalent

CAUTION: Federal (U.S.A.) law prohibits dispensing without prescription.
SINGLE DOSE VIAL

MERCK SHARP & DOHME
DIVISION OF MERCK & CO. INC.
WEST POINT, PA. 19486, U.S.A.

Bottle 4

#228-1

NDC 0069-5460-74   9249

Vistaril®
hydroxyzine
hydrochloride

50 mg / ml

10 ml

INTRAMUSCULAR SOLUTION

CAUTION: Federal law prohibits
dispensing without prescription.

READ ACCOMPANYING
PROFESSIONAL
INFORMATION

Each ml contains **50 mg** of hydroxyzine hydrochloride, 0.9%
benzyl alcohol and sodium hydroxide to adjust to optimum pH.

USUAL ADULT DOSE
Intramuscularly: 25—100 mg
stat; repeat every 4 to 6 hours,
as needed.

To avoid discoloration,
protect from prolonged
exposure to light.

U S Pat No. 2 899 436

P F I Z E R   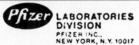 **LABORATORIES
DIVISION**
PFIZER INC.,
NEW YORK, N.Y. 10017   **P F I Z E R**

10-1111-00-9
B-5344A

MADE IN U.S.A.

SIMKINS
7

Bottle 5

WORKSHEET: EXERCISE IN READING DRUG BOTTLE LABELS

Find each of the items listed on the sample drug bottle labels found on pages 26, 27 and 28.

	Bottle 1	Bottle 2	Bottle 3	Bottle 4	Bottle 5
1. Trade name	Compazine Spansule	Ilosone Liquid	Tranxene	Sodium Edecrin	
2. Generic name or nonproprietary name	Prochlorperazine	Erythromycin Estolate Oral Suspension USP	Clorazepate dipotassium	Ethacrynate sodium	
3. Strength	30 mg	125 mg	3.75 mg	50 mg	
4. Total contents of bottle, i.e., number of capsules	50 caps	16 fl oz (1pt) (473 mL)	100 Cap	50 cc	
5. Usual dosage	1 cap per day. Accomp times folder for complete infor.	See Accompanying literature for dosage	See package enclosure for dosage + prescribing Info.		
6. Special precautions	Use safety Closures when dispensing this product unless otherwise directed by Physician or Requested	Federal USA law prohibits dispensing w/out Prescription	Federal USA Prohibits dispensing w/out Prescription		

WORKSHEET: EXERCISE IN READING DRUG BOTTLE LABELS (continued)

	Bottle 1	Bottle 2	Bottle 3	Bottle 4	Bottle 5
7. Mixing instructions if applicable					
8. Route of administration					
9. Type of drug					
10. Special storage instructions					
11. Manufacturer's name					
12. Expiration date					

ANSWER SHEET: EXERCISE IN READING DRUG BOTTLE LABELS

	Bottle 1	Bottle 2	Bottle 3	Bottle 4	Bottle 5
1. Trade name	Compazine® Spansule®	Ilosone® Liquid	Tranxene®	Sodium Edecrin®	Vistaril®
2. Generic name or nonproprietary name	prochlorperazine	erythromycin estolate oral suspension, USP	clorazepate dipotassium	ethacrynate sodium	hydroxyzine hydrochloride
3. Strength	30 mg capsules	125 mg per 5 ml	3.75 mg	50 mg	50 mg per ml
4. Total contents of bottle, i.e., number of capsules	50 capsules	16 Fl oz (1 pt) (473 ml)	100 capsules	50 mg of dry powdered drug. Single dose vial	10 ml
5. Usual dosage	1 capsule daily. See accompanying folder for complete prescribing information.	See accompanying literature for dosage	See package enclosure for dosage and full prescribing information.	See accompanying circular.	Intramuscularly 25–100 mg stat; repeat every 4 to 6 hours, as needed.
6. Special precautions	Federal law prohibits dispensing without prescription. Use safety closures when dispensing.	Federal law prohibits dispensing without prescription.	Federal (U.S.A.) law prohibits dispensing without prescription. Controlled substance schedule IV	Federal (U.S.A.) law prohibits dispensing without prescription.	Caution: Federal law prohibits dispensing without prescription. To avoid discoloration, protect from prolonged exposure to light.

ANSWER SHEET: EXERCISE IN READING DRUG BOTTLE LABELS (*continued*)

	Bottle 1	Bottle 2	Bottle 3	Bottle 4	Bottle 5
7. Mixing instructions if applicable	—	Shake well before using. (This drug is a suspension. The drug settles to the bottom.)	—	To reconstitute, add 50 ml of 5% dextrose injection or sodium chloride injection for slow intravenous injection.	—
8. Route of administration	Oral	Oral	Oral	Intravenous injection	For intramuscular use only.
9. Type of drug	Sustained release capsule	Oral suspension	Capsule	Powder to be reconstituted	Liquid preparation for IM injection. Intramuscular solution.
10. Special storage instructions	Store at controlled room temperature.	Keep tightly closed. Refrigerate to maintain optimum taste.	Keep bottle tightly closed. Dispense in a USP tight container.	Discard unused solution after 24 hours.	Store below 86°F (30°C)
11. Manufacturer's name	Smith Kline & French (SK&F) Laboratories	Dista Products Co. a Division of Eli Lilly & Co. Inc.	Abbott Pharmaceuticals Inc.	Merck Sharp & Dohme	Pfizer Laboratories Division
12. Expiration date	NO EXPIRATION DATE IS GIVEN ON THESE LABELS BECAUSE THEY WERE "SAMPLE" LABELS *REMEMBER TO CHECK THE EXPIRATION DATE!*				

Feb 16 84

$$\frac{D}{H} \times V$$

D = Dose Dr. Order

V = Vehicle how it comes

H = Drug dose on hand

6 Working Dosage Problems

OBJECTIVES

After completing this chapter, the student will be able to:

1. *Work dosage problems, using either a formula or ratio and proportion.*
2. *Identify the dosage strength of a drug from the drug label and use this information to work the dosage problem.*
3. *Identify the drug order on a physician's order sheet.*
4. *Shade syringes and medication cup to the correct dosage measurement.*

Medications are prepared in either liquid, solid, or gaseous form. Medications may be administered by a number of different routes: the enteral (oral, rectal); the parenteral (injections); and the percutaneous (sublingual, inhalation). The nurse must be certain that the dosage form of the medication is being administered by the correct route. The form (or vehicle) in which the medication is prepared determines the route by which it can be administered. Read the label carefully for the route of administration.

A given concentration of drug is put into a tablet, a capsule, or a liquid vehicle by the pharmaceutical company (to be administered to the person needing the medication).

The physician will write an order for the medication in a prescription, or on the physician's order sheet, for the drug to be administered by the nurse. The drug is then ordered from the hospital pharmacy for administration. The medication may be sent to the nursing unit as a unit-dose preparation, or the nurse may have to get it from a stock supply of drugs. In either case, the nurse must check carefully for the correct drug, dosage, and route. She/he will then administer it to the right patient on time.

If the preparation is not packaged in the correct dosage strength, ordered by the physician, the nurse must calculate the number of tablets, capsules, or the amount of the liquid containing the prescribed dose.

Either a formula or a proportion may be used to determine the amount of medication containing the prescribed dosage. Choose the method that you find easiest for you. Do not try to use both methods but *learn one method thoroughly!*

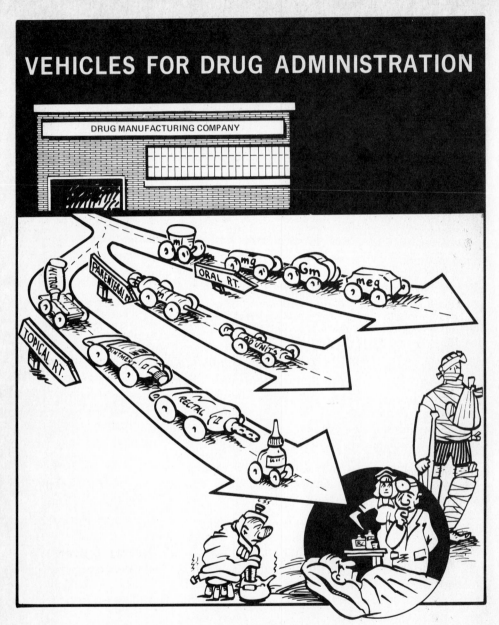

Figure 6.1 Vehicles for Drug Administration.

METHOD I—SUGGESTED FORMULA

$$\frac{\text{Dose ordered}}{\text{Drug strength on hand}} \times (\text{tablet, cap-sule, liquid})^{\text{Vehicle}} = \text{Amount to give}$$

$$\frac{D}{H} \times V = \text{Amount to give}$$

The desired drug dose = Amount of drug ordered by the physician.
Drug strength on hand = Drug dosage from which to obtain the ordered dose.
Vehicle = Capsule, tablet, or liquid containing the dose on hand.

Example 1

The physician orders Keflex 750 mg.

Step 1: Look at the medicine bottle label (Fig. 6.2).
Each capsule of Keflex contains 250 mg.
Both the drug ordered and the drug on hand are in the same unit of measure: milligrams

Step 2: Substitute into the formula

$$\frac{D}{H} \times V = \text{Amount to give}$$

$$\frac{\text{Dose ordered}}{\text{Strength on hand}} \qquad \frac{750 \text{ mg}}{250 \text{ mg}} \times 1 \text{ capsule} = G$$

$$\frac{\overset{3}{\cancel{750}}}{\underset{1}{\cancel{250}}} \times 1 \text{ capsule} = 3 \text{ capsules of Keflex} \atop 250 \text{ mg each}$$

Be sure to label each number in the formula.
You may work the problem without canceling if you wish.

Step 3: Think: "I have 250 mg in one capsule; there are 750 mg in 3 capsules."
Ask yourself if your answer is logical. Check your answer by an alternate method of reasoning: 250 mg × 3 = 750 mg.

Step 4: Administer 3 capsules to the patient.

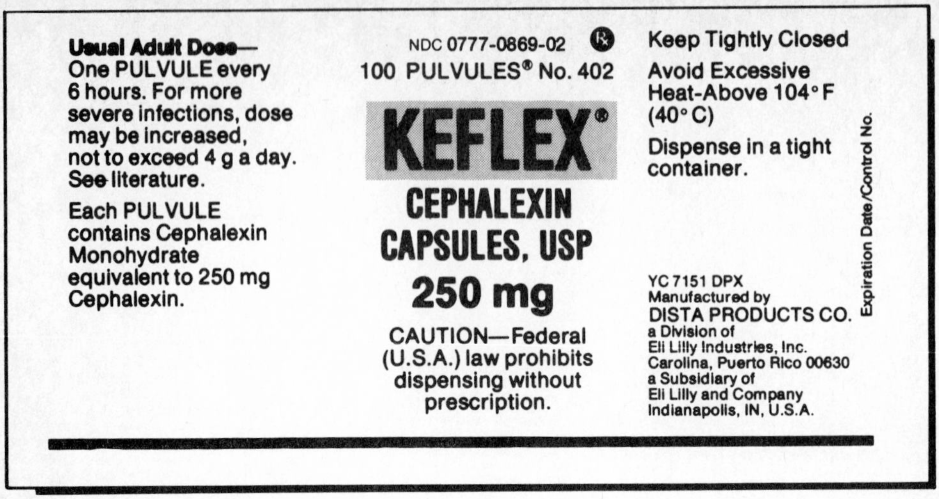

Figure 6.2

METHOD II—SUGGESTED RATIO AND PROPORTION

Remember to compare like things to like things. Set up a ratio of information on the label for one part of the proportion and the dosage desired as the other ratio and the other part of the proportion. Compare drug to vehicle on hand to drug to vehicle desired.

Drug label   Drug desired
information
Drug : Vehicle   Drug : Amount of Vehicle to give
Strength on hand : Vehicle :: Dosage ordered : Amount to give

Example 1

The physician orders Keflex 0.5 gm (Fig. 6.2)

Step 1: Look at the label. Each capsule contains 250 mg of Keflex. Convert so that desired dosage and the available dosage is in the same unit of measure. The order is in grams, the available capsules are in milligrams. Convert to the available unit.

$$0.5 \text{ gm} = 500 \text{ mg}$$

Step 2: Substitute into the formula.

Strength on hand : Vehicle : : Dose ordered : Amount to give
H : V : :   D :   G

Multiply the means together and the extremes together. Label all parts of the proportion.

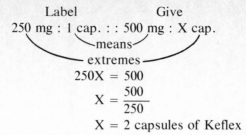

$$\text{250 mg : 1 cap. : : 500 mg : X cap.}$$
$$\overbrace{\qquad\qquad}^{\text{means}}$$
$$\text{extremes}$$

$$250X = 500$$
$$X = \frac{500}{250}$$
$$X = 2 \text{ capsules of Keflex}$$

You may set up the proportion as a fraction.

Cross multiply
$$\frac{250 \text{ mg}}{1 \text{ cap.}} : : \frac{500 \text{ mg}}{X \text{ cap.}}$$
$$250X = 500$$
$$X = \frac{500}{250}$$
$$X = 2 \text{ capsules}$$

Step 3: *ALWAYS* check your arithmetic, preferably by an alternate method to avoid medication errors.

For example, in your mind ask: Do two 250 mg capsules equal 500 mg?

$$\frac{250 \text{ mg}}{\frac{250 \text{ mg}}{500 \text{ mg}}} \quad \text{or} \quad \frac{250}{\frac{X\ 2}{500}}$$

If the arithmetic is correct when you double-checked your math,

Step 4: Administer the *correct* dosage.

You can never be too cautious with medicine.

Example 2

The physician orders Benadryl 50 mg.

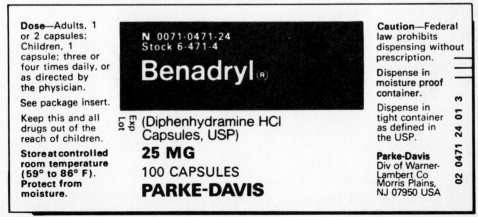

Figure 6.3

Set up your dosage problem by the method you prefer, using the four steps listed to prepare to administer the medication. After you have tried to work the problem, check your work with the example.

$$\frac{D}{H} \times V = G \text{ (Dose to give)}$$

$$\frac{50 \text{ mg}}{25 \text{ mg}} \times 1 \text{ cap.} = 2 \text{ capsules of Benadryl to be administered}$$

In this problem, the units were the same so you didn't have to convert.

Strength on hand	:	Vehicle	: :	Dose ordered	:	Amount to give
H	:	V	: :	D	:	G
25 mg	:	1 cap.	: :	50 mg	:	X cap.

$$25X = 50$$
$$X = 2 \text{ capsules of Benadryl to be administered}$$

Remember the vehicle contains the required dosage you are to administer (capsules, tablets, milliliters, drams, teaspoons, ounces, etc.). You do not administer milligrams or grams. You administer X number of milligrams or grams or units in some type of vehicle (tablet, capsule, or liquid).

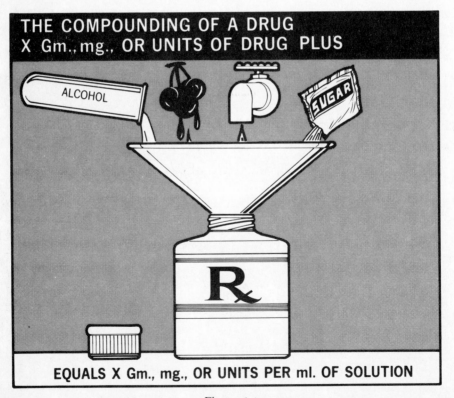

THE COMPOUNDING OF A DRUG X Gm., mg., OR UNITS OF DRUG PLUS

ALCOHOL   SUGAR

Rx

EQUALS X Gm., mg., OR UNITS PER ml. OF SOLUTION

Figure 6.4

Example 3

The physician orders Depakene (valproic acid) 500 mg.

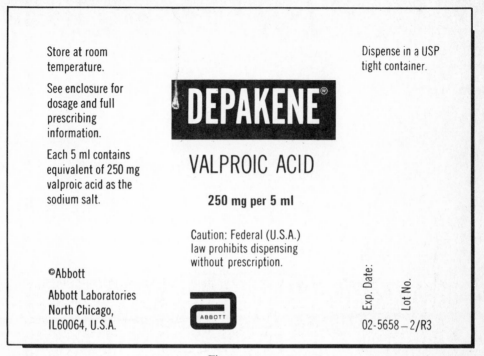

Store at room temperature.

See enclosure for dosage and full prescribing information.

Each 5 ml contains equivalent of 250 mg valproic acid as the sodium salt.

©Abbott

Abbott Laboratories
North Chicago,
IL60064, U.S.A.

Dispense in a USP tight container.

DEPAKENE®

VALPROIC ACID

250 mg per 5 ml

Caution: Federal (U.S.A.) law prohibits dispensing without prescription.

Exp. Date:

Lot No.

02-5658 – 2/R3

Figure 6.5

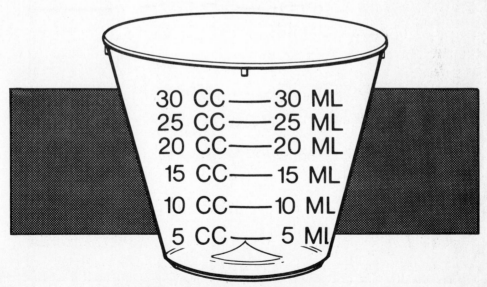

30 CC —— 30 ML
25 CC —— 25 ML
20 CC —— 20 ML
15 CC —— 15 ML
10 CC —— 10 ML
5 CC —— 5 ML

Figure 6.6   Fill medicine glass to correct dosage.

Set up your dosage problem by the method you prefer. Work using the four steps outlined.

Formula:

$$\frac{D}{H} \times V = \text{Dose to be administered}$$

$$\frac{\overset{2}{\cancel{500}} \text{mg}}{\underset{1}{\cancel{250}} \text{mg}} \times 5 \text{ ml} = 10 \text{ ml of Depakene Syrup to be administered}$$

Ratio Method:

$$\begin{array}{cccccc} \text{H} & : & \text{V} & :: & \text{D} & : & \text{G} \\ 250 \text{ mg} & : & 5 \text{ ml} & :: & 500 \text{ mg} & : & \text{X ml} \end{array} \quad \text{or} \quad \frac{250 \text{ mg}}{5 \text{ ml}} :: \frac{500 \text{ mg}}{\text{X ml}}$$

$$250\text{X} = 2500 \qquad\qquad\qquad \text{cross multiply}$$

$$\text{X} = \frac{2500}{250}$$

$$\text{X} = 10 \text{ ml of Depakene}$$

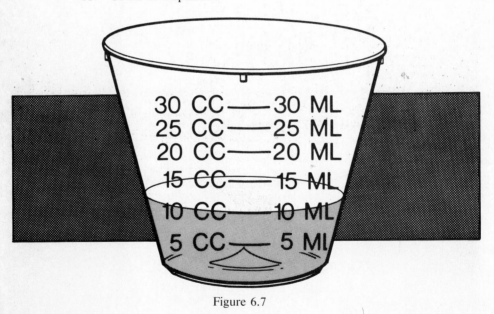

Figure 6.7

In this problem the vehicle is a liquid. The dosage strength, 250 mg, is contained in 5 milliliters of syrup. The patient is to receive 500 milligrams. The correct dosage for this patient is 10 milliliters of Depakene Syrup.

Using the physicians order sheet (Fig. 6.8) and the drug labels (Figs. 6.9 to 6.17) calculate the correct dosage to be administered. Shade the medicine glass or syringe as indicated for each problem.

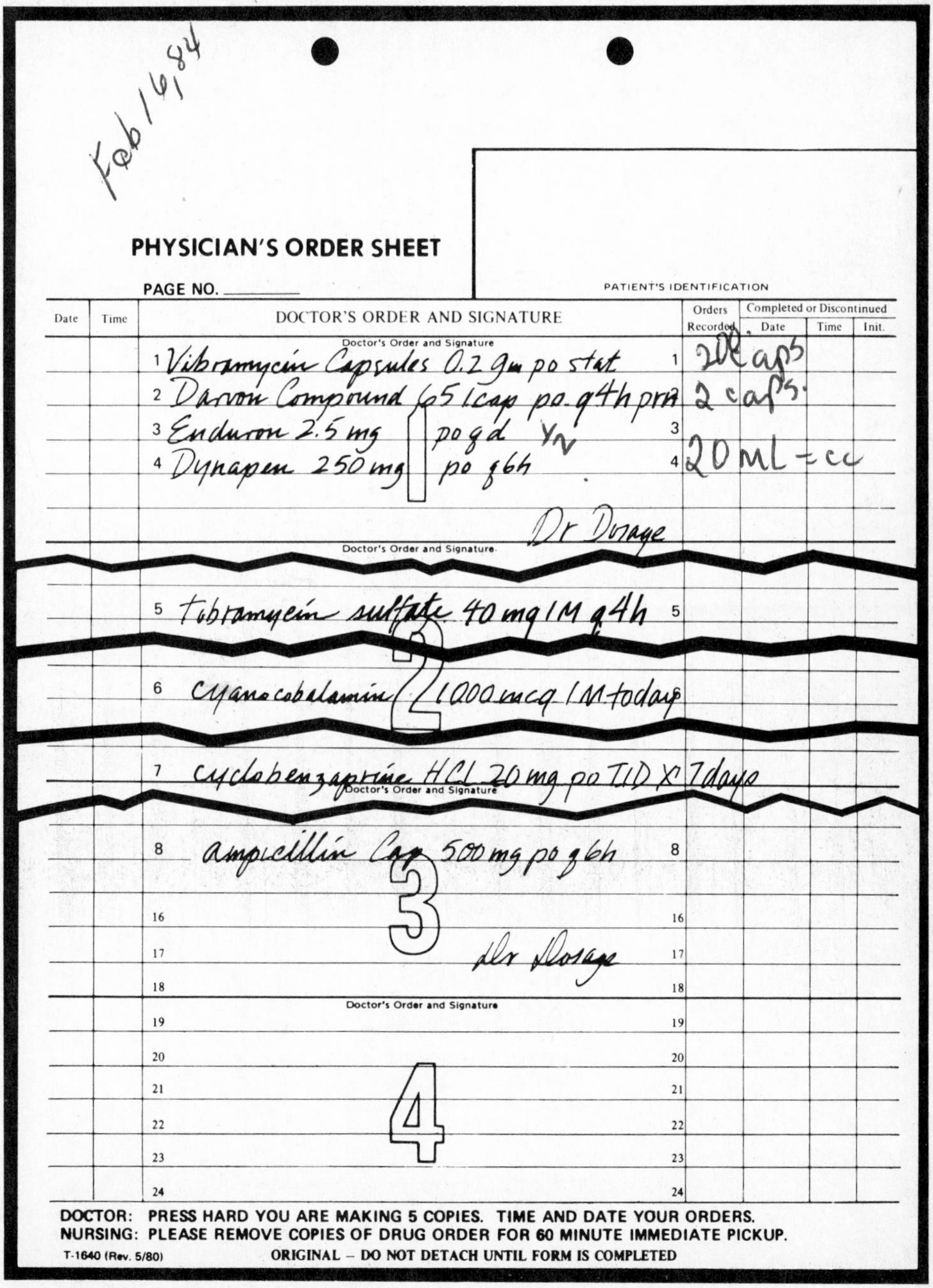

Feb/16/84

PHYSICIAN'S ORDER SHEET

PAGE NO. _____

PATIENT'S IDENTIFICATION

Date	Time	DOCTOR'S ORDER AND SIGNATURE	Orders Recorded	Completed or Discontinued		
				Date	Time	Init.
		Doctor's Order and Signature				
		1 Vibramycin Capsules 0.2 gm po stat	1	2 caps		
		2 Darvon Compound 65 1cap po. q4h prn	2	2 caps.		
		3 Enduron 2.5 mg po qd ½	3			
		4 Dynapen 250 mg po q6h	4	20 mL = cc		
		Dr Dosage				
		Doctor's Order and Signature				
		5 Tobramycin sulfate 40 mg IM q4h	5			
		6 Cyanocobalamin 1000 mcg IM today				
		7 cyclobenzaprine HCl 20 mg po TID x 7days				
		Doctor's Order and Signature				
		8 ampicillin Cap 500 mg po q6h	8			
		16	16			
		17 Dr Dosage	17			
		18	18			
		Doctor's Order and Signature				
		19	19			
		20	20			
		21	21			
		22	22			
		23	23			
		24	24			

DOCTOR: PRESS HARD YOU ARE MAKING 5 COPIES. TIME AND DATE YOUR ORDERS.
NURSING: PLEASE REMOVE COPIES OF DRUG ORDER FOR 60 MINUTE IMMEDIATE PICKUP.
T-1640 (Rev. 5/80)   ORIGINAL – DO NOT DETACH UNTIL FORM IS COMPLETED

Figure 6.8

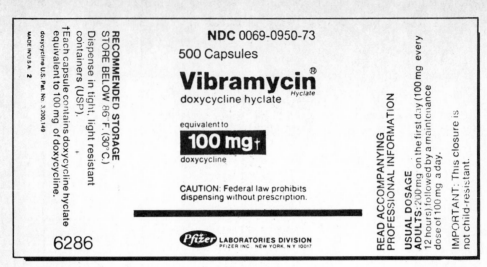

Figure 6.9

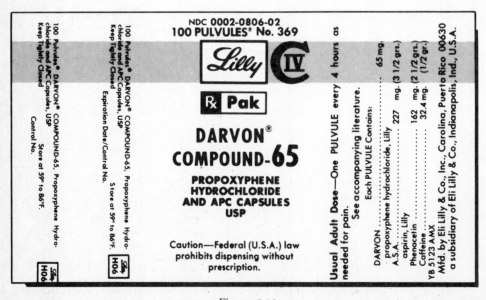

Figure 6.10

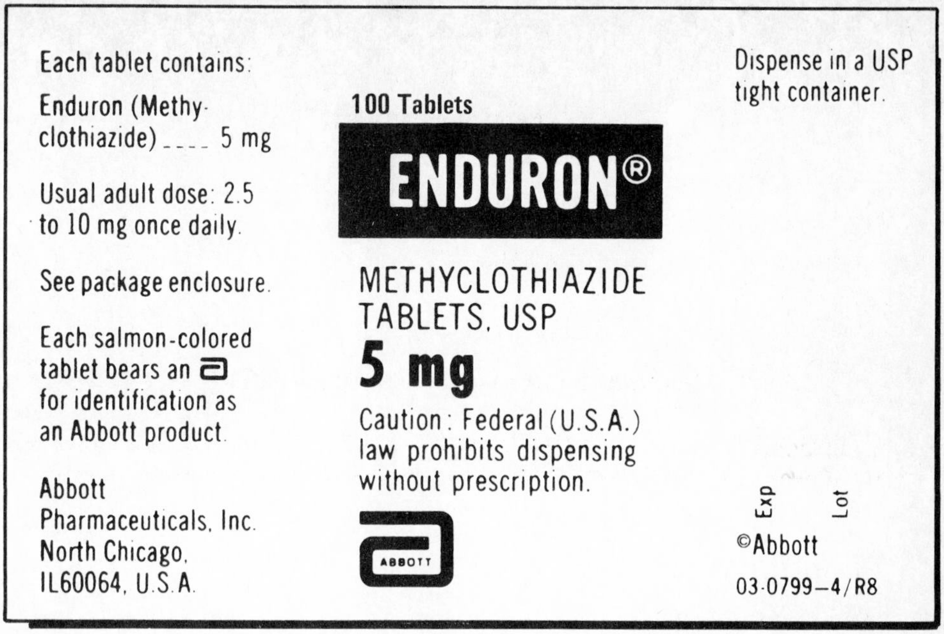

Each tablet contains:

Enduron (Methy-
clothiazide) ____ 5 mg

Usual adult dose: 2.5
to 10 mg once daily.

See package enclosure.

Each salmon-colored
tablet bears an ⊃
for identification as
an Abbott product.

Abbott
Pharmaceuticals, Inc.
North Chicago,
IL60064, U.S.A.

100 Tablets

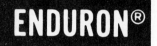

ENDURON®

METHYCLOTHIAZIDE
TABLETS, USP

5 mg

Caution: Federal (U.S.A.)
law prohibits dispensing
without prescription.

Dispense in a USP
tight container.

Exp   Lot

©Abbott

03-0799−4/R8

Figure 6.11

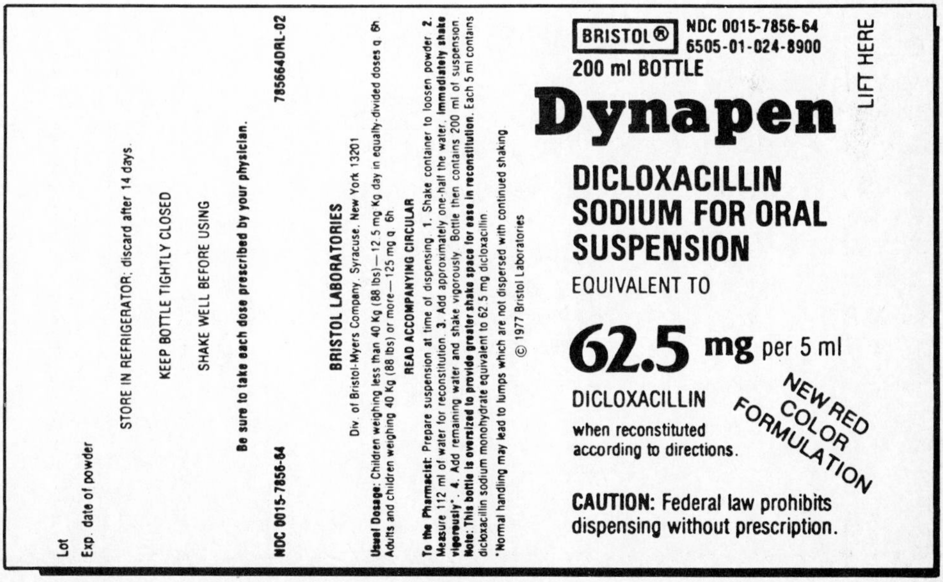

Lot
Exp. date of powder

STORE IN REFRIGERATOR: discard after 14 days.

KEEP BOTTLE TIGHTLY CLOSED

SHAKE WELL BEFORE USING

Be sure to take each dose prescribed by your physician.

785664ORL-02

BRISTOL LABORATORIES

Div. of Bristol-Myers Company. Syracuse, New York 13201

Usual Dosage: Children weighing less than 40 Kg (88 lbs)—12.5 mg Kg day in equally-divided doses q 6h
Adults and children weighing 40 Kg (88 lbs) or more—125 mg q 6h

READ ACCOMPANYING CIRCULAR

To the Pharmacist: Prepare suspension at time of dispensing. 1. Shake container to loosen powder. 2. Measure 112 ml of water for reconstitution. 3. Add approximately one-half the water. **Immediately shake vigorously*.** 4. Add remaining water and shake vigorously. Bottle then contains 200 ml of suspension. **Note:** This bottle is oversized to provide greater shake space for ease in reconstitution. Each 5 ml contains dicloxacillin sodium monohydrate equivalent to 62.5 mg dicloxacillin
*Normal handling may lead to lumps which are not dispersed with continued shaking.

© 1977 Bristol Laboratories

NDC 0015-7856-64

BRISTOL®   NDC 0015-7856-64
                6505-01-024-8900

200 ml BOTTLE

LIFT HERE

Dynapen

**DICLOXACILLIN
SODIUM FOR ORAL
SUSPENSION**

EQUIVALENT TO

62.5 mg per 5 ml

DICLOXACILLIN

when reconstituted
according to directions.

NEW RED
COLOR
FORMULATION

CAUTION: Federal law prohibits
dispensing without prescription.

Figure 6.12

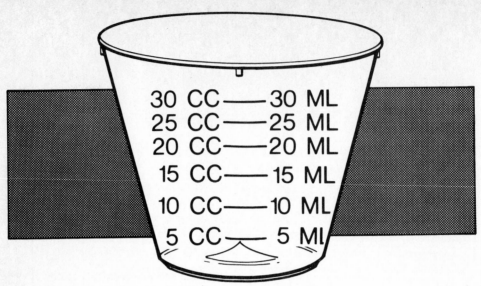

Figure 6.13 Fill medicine glass to correct dosage.

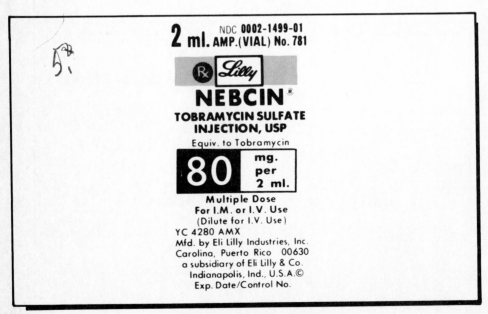

Figure 6.14 (See Fig. 6.18).

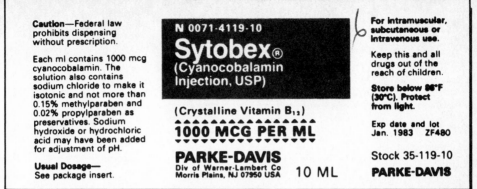

Caution—Federal law prohibits dispensing without prescription.

Each ml contains 1000 mcg cyanocobalamin. The solution also contains sodium chloride to make it isotonic and not more than 0.15% methylparaben and 0.02% propylparaben as preservatives. Sodium hydroxide or hydrochloric acid may have been added for adjustment of pH.

Usual Dosage— See package insert.

N 0071-4119-10
Sytobex®
(Cyanocobalamin Injection, USP)

(Crystalline Vitamin B₁₂)
1000 MCG PER ML

PARKE-DAVIS
Div of Warner-Lambert Co
Morris Plains, NJ 07950 USA   10 ML

For intramuscular, subcutaneous or intravenous use.

Keep this and all drugs out of the reach of children.

Store below 86°F (30°C). Protect from light.

Exp date and lot Jan. 1983   ZF480

Stock 35-119-10

PARKE-DAVIS

Figure 6.15 (See Fig. 6.19).

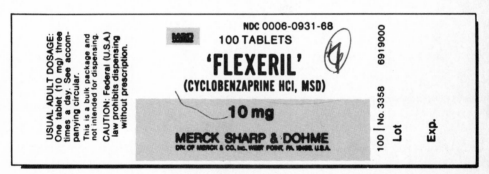

USUAL ADULT DOSAGE: One tablet (10 mg) three times a day. See accompanying circular.

This is a bulk package and not intended for dispensing.

CAUTION: Federal (U.S.A.) law prohibits dispensing without prescription.

NDC 0006-0931-68
100 TABLETS

'FLEXERIL'
(CYCLOBENZAPRINE HCl, MSD)

10 mg

MERCK SHARP & DOHME
DIV. OF MERCK & CO., Inc., WEST POINT, PA. 19486. U.S.A.

100 | No. 3358   6919000

Lot   Exp.

Figure 6.16

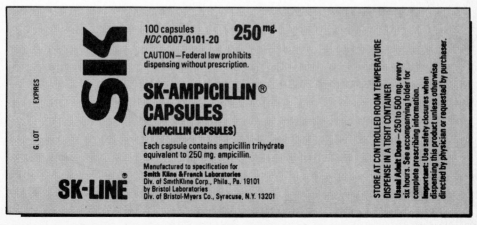

SK

100 capsules
NDC 0007-0101-20   **250 mg.**

CAUTION—Federal law prohibits dispensing without prescription.

SK-AMPICILLIN®
CAPSULES

(AMPICILLIN CAPSULES)

Each capsule contains ampicillin trihydrate equivalent to 250 mg. ampicillin.

Manufactured to specification for
Smith Kline &French Laboratories
Div. of SmithKline Corp., Phila., Pa. 19101
by Bristol Laboratories
Div. of Bristol-Myers Co., Syracuse, N.Y. 13201

SK-LINE®

G. LOT   EXPIRES

STORE AT CONTROLLED ROOM TEMPERATURE
DISPENSE IN A TIGHT CONTAINER
Usual Adult Dose—250 to 500 mg. every six hours. See accompanying folder for complete prescribing information.
Important: Use safety closures when dispensing this product unless otherwise directed by physician or requested by purchaser.

Figure 6.17

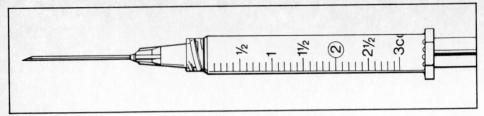

Figure 6.18   Shade syringe to correct line.

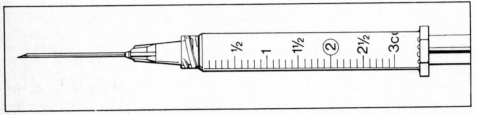

Figure 6.19   Shade syringe to correct line.

ANSWERS: DOSAGE PROBLEMS

1. $\dfrac{D}{H} \times V = G$ Order 0.2 gm = 200 mg

   $$\dfrac{\overset{2}{\cancel{200}} \text{ mg}}{\underset{1}{\cancel{100}} \text{ mg}} \times 1 \text{ cap.} = 2 \text{ capsules of Vibromycin}$$

2. Darvon Compound-65 is a compound of Darvon 65 mg, aspirin 227 mg, phenacetin 162 mg, caffeine 32.4 mg. The order is for 1 capsule. Give 1 capsule; there is no problem to work. Just be sure you give the correct medicine. There are several different Darvon preparations.

3.   H :   V ::   D : G
   5 mg :   1 tablet: : 2.5 mg : X tab.
             5X = 2.5
             $X = \dfrac{2.5}{5}$
             X = 0.5 or ½ tablet of Enduron

   Note this tablet is grooved (scored), so it may be cut in half.

4. $\dfrac{D}{H} \times V = G$

$\dfrac{\overset{4}{\cancel{250}}\text{ mg}}{\underset{1}{\cancel{62.5}}\text{ mg}} \times 5\text{ ml} = 20\text{ ml of Dynapen}$

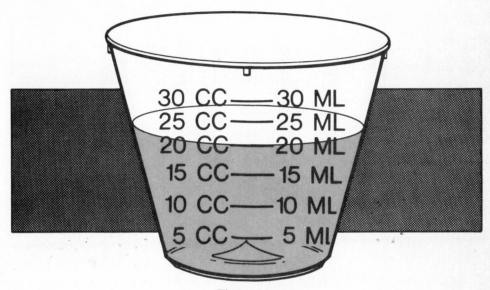

Figure 6.20

Dynapen is a suspension 62.5 mg of dicloxacillin per 5 ml. Observe that the instructions on the label say "Shake well before using." Be certain to read the label for special administration instructions.

5. $\quad$ H $\quad$: $\quad$ V :: $\quad$ D $\quad$: G
$\quad$ 80 mg $\quad$: 2 ml : 40 mg : X ml
$\qquad$ 80X = 80
$\qquad$ X = 1 ml tobramycin

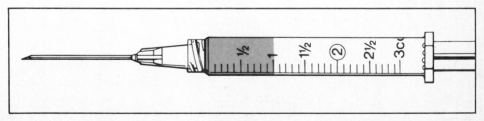

Figure 6.21

6. $\dfrac{D}{H} \times V = $ Dose

$$\dfrac{1000 \text{ mcg}}{1000 \text{ mcg}} \times 1 \text{ ml} = 1 \text{ ml}$$

This problem doesn't need to be worked since the desired dose and the "have" dose are the same.

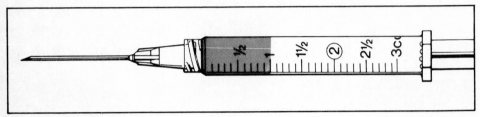

Figure 6.22

7. $\dfrac{H}{V} :: \dfrac{D}{G}$

$$\dfrac{10 \text{ mg}}{1 \text{ tab.}} :: \dfrac{20 \text{ mg}}{X \text{ tab.}}$$

$$10X = 20$$
$$X = 2 \text{ tab. of cyclobenzaprine HCl}$$

Look carefully at the spelling of the name of the drug you are to give. Be certain you have the correct drug, names are frequently very similar.

8. $\dfrac{D}{H} \times V = D$

$$\dfrac{\overset{2}{\cancel{500}} \text{ mg}}{\underset{1}{\cancel{250}} \text{ mg}} \times 1 \text{ cap.} = 2 \text{ capsules ampicillin}$$

7   Units and Milliequivalents

OBJECTIVES

After studying the content of this chapter, the student will be able to:

1. *Define unit.*
2. *Define milliequivalent.*
3. *Use a formula or proportion to solve dosage problems of drugs ordered in units.*
4. *Use a formula or proportion to solve dosage problems of drugs ordered in milliequivalents.*

Dosage problems involving drugs which are measured in units other than metric or apothecaries' system units are worked by the same formulas used for other dosage problems. The units or milliequivalents of drug use tablets, capsules, or milliliters of liquid as the vehicle. Work problems using the same formula or proportion that you have been using, substituting the units or milliequivalents into the dose ordered and strength on hand positions.

PROBLEMS USING UNITS AND MILLIEQUIVALENTS

A unit of drug is one that cannot be analyzed by chemical means. The drug is standardized by its effect on laboratory animals under controlled conditions. The strength is determined by the amount of drug required to bring about a desired effect in a laboratory animal. The strength of hormones and vitamins is measured in units. The abbreviation for unit is U.

The physician orders penicillin G 600,000 units. The vial has been reconstituted to 500,000 units/1 ml. How much solution should be given?

$$\frac{D}{H} \times V = G$$

Method #1 $\dfrac{600,000U}{500,000U} \times 1\ ml = \dfrac{6}{5} = 1.18$ or 1.2 ml of penicillin G

Method #2   H :   V   : :   D   : G
                 500,000U : 1 ml : : 600,000U : X ml
                     500,000 X = 600,000
                            X = 600,000 ÷ 500,000
                            X = 1.18 or 1.2 ml of penicillin G

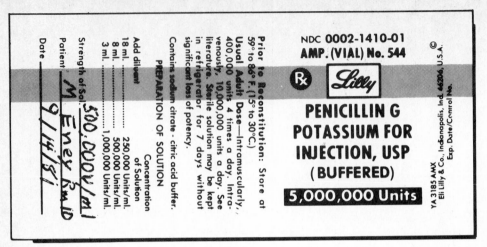

Figure 7.1

An equivalent is the unit of measure for chemical combining activity of an electrolyte. The chemical combining activity is based upon the number of available ionic charges (cations, anions) in solution. The concentration of electrolytes in biology is small and is therefore expressed as milliequivalents, 1/1000 of an equivalent. One milliequivalent of any ion can react completely with one milliequivalent of any cation. The abbreviation for milliequivalent is mEq. Drugs used to maintain the body's electrolyte balance are usually measured in milliequivalents.

The physician orders 80 mEq of ammonium chloride to be added to 1000 ml of D_5W. The strength on hand is 100 mEq/20 ml. How much ammonium chloride must be added to the IV?

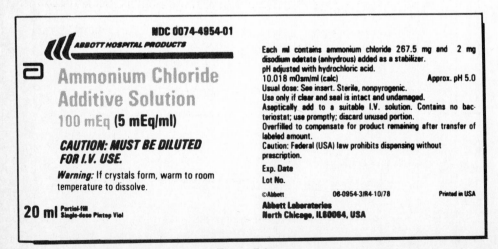

Figure 7.2

$$\frac{D}{H} \times V = G$$

$$\frac{\cancel{80}\,\text{mEq}}{\cancel{100}\,\text{mEq}} \times \overset{2}{\cancel{20}}\,\text{ml} = 16\,\text{ml of ammonium chloride}$$

H : V :: D : G

100 mEq : 20 ml : : 80 mEq : X ml

100X = 1600

X = 16 ml of ammonium chloride

UNITS AND MILLIEQUIVALENTS: PROBLEMS

1. Give 5,000 U of Heparin. Label reads 10,000 U per ml.

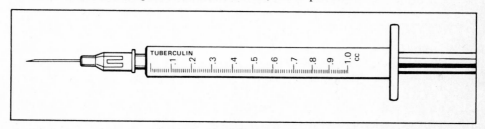

Figure 7.3

2. Give 7,000 U of Heparin. Label reads 10,000 U per ml.

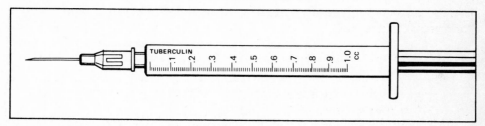

Figure 7.4

3. Give 500,000 U of Bicillin. Label reads 1,000,000 U per 5 ml.

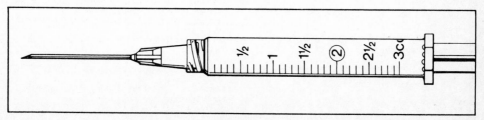

Figure 7.5

4. The doctor orders 150 U of a drug. Given a vial containing 750 U per 5 ml. How much will you give?

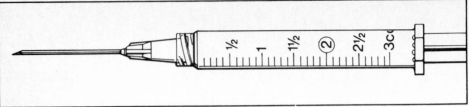

Figure 7.6

5. Give 50,000 U of sodium penicillin G from a multiple-dose vial containing 1,000,000 U per 10 ml.

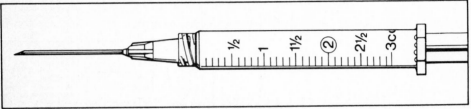

Figure 7.7

6. You are told to add 30 mEq of potassium chloride to an IV. The label on the potassium chloride vial reads 40 mEq/10 ml. How many ml will you add?

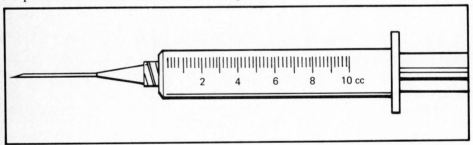

Figure 7.8

7. Add 20 U of Syntocinon to an IV. Syntocinon is supplied in 1 ml ampules 5 U/ml.

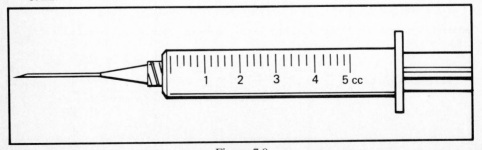

Figure 7.9

8. Give 15 mEq of potassium gluconate. Each tablet contains 5 mEq. How many tablets would you give?

ANSWERS TO UNITS AND EQUIVALENTS MILLI PROBLEMS:

1. *Method #1*

$$\frac{5000 \text{ U}}{10000 \text{ U}} \times 1 \text{ ml} = \frac{5000}{10000} = 0.5 \text{ ml of heparin}$$

Method #2

10000 U : 1 ml = 5000 U : X ml
    10000 X = 5000
        X = 5000 ÷ 10000
        X = 0.5 ml of heparin

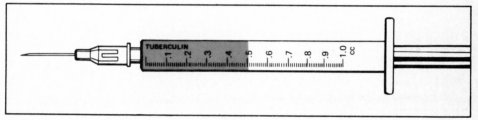

Figure 7.10

2. *Method #1*

$$\frac{7000 \text{ U}}{10000 \text{ U}} \times 1 \text{ ml} = \frac{7000}{10000} = 0.7 \text{ ml of heparin}$$

Method #2

10000 U : 1 ml = 7000 : X ml
    10000 X = 7000
        X = 7000 ÷ 10000
        X = 0.7 ml of heparin

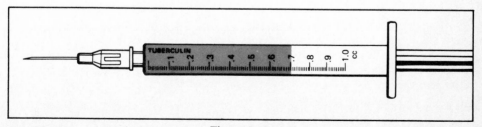

Figure 7.11

3. *Method #1*

$$\frac{500,000 \text{ U}}{1,000,000 \text{ U}} \times 5 \text{ ml} = \frac{2,500,000}{1,000,000} = 2.5 \text{ ml of Bicillin}$$

Method #2

1,000,000 U : 5 ml = 5,000,000 : X ml
   1,000,000 X = 2,500,000
      X = 2,500,000 ÷ 1,000,000
      X = 2.5 ml of Bicillin

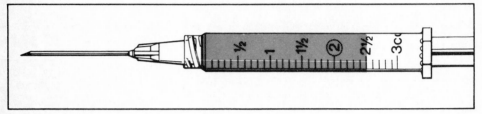

Figure 7.12

4. *Method #1*

$$\frac{150 \text{ U}}{750 \text{ U}} \times 5 \text{ ml} = \frac{750}{750} = 1 \text{ ml of the drug ordered}$$

Method #2

750 U : 5 ml : : 150 U : X ml
   750 X = 750
     X = 1 ml of the drug ordered

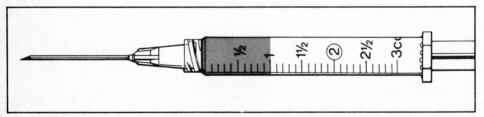

Figure 7.13

5. *Method #1*

$$\frac{50,000 \text{ U}}{1,000,000 \text{ U}} \times 10 \text{ ml} = \frac{500,000}{1,000,000} = 0.5 \text{ ml of penicillin G}$$

Method #2

1,000,000 U : 10 ml = 50,000 U : X ml
  1,000,000 X = 500,000
         X = 500,000 ÷ 1,000,000
         X = 0.5 ml of penicillin G

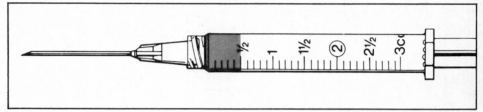

Figure 7.14

6. *Method #1*

$$\frac{30 \text{ mEq}}{40 \text{ mEq}} \times 10 \text{ ml} = \frac{300}{40} = 7.5 \text{ ml of KCl}$$

Method #2

40 mEq : 10 ml : : 30 mEq : X ml
    40 X = 300
     X = 300 ÷ 40
     X = 7.5 ml of KCl

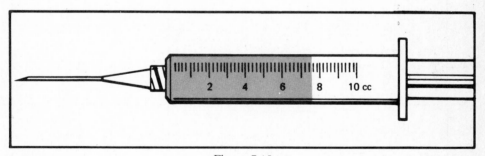

Figure 7.15

7. *Method #1*

$$\frac{20 \text{ U}}{5 \text{ U}} \times 1 \text{ ml} = \frac{20}{5} = 4 \text{ ml of Syntocinon}$$

Method #2

5 U : 1 ml : : 20 U : X ml
    5 X = 20
     X = 4 ml of Syntocinon

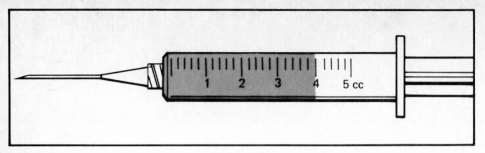

Figure 7.16

8. *Method #1*

$$\frac{15 \text{ mEq}}{5 \text{ mEq}} \times 1 \text{ tab.} = \frac{15}{5} = 3 \text{ tab. of potassium gluconate}$$

Method #2

5 mEq : 1 tab. : : 15 mEq : X tab.
$$5 X = 15$$
$$X = 15 \div 5$$
$$X = 3 \text{ tab. of potassium gluconate}$$

8   Insulin Administration

OBJECTIVES

After completing this chapter, the student will be able to:

1. *Choose the correct insulin preparation.*
2. *Select the correct syringe for preparing the insulin dosage.*
3. *Shade the appropriate syringe to the correct dosage.*
4. *State the three things necessary for safe insulin preparation.*

Insulin is a hormone necessary for carbohydrate metabolism in the body. It is produced in the pancreas. Insulin is prepared in so many units per ml. There is a trend to use only 100 unit insulin to cut down on dosage errors. However, insulin is still manufactured in other strengths—20 units/ml, 40 units/ml, and 500 units/ml. The potency of the insulin does not alter the strength of the unit.

To administer insulin, use an insulin syringe calibrated in units the same as the strength of the insulin being used. In other words, you would use a U-40 (Unit 40) insulin syringe with 40 unit/cc insulin, a U-100 insulin syringe with 100 unit/cc insulin. *ALWAYS* use the correct syringe for the strength insulin to be used. *DO NOT* try to interchange syringes. The Food and Drug Administration decertified U-80 insulin (80 Units per ml) March 24, 1980.

Be careful to choose the right kind of insulin. There are different insulin preparations; some are short acting and must be given before each meal. Others have a medium range action time and others are long acting. In the illustration there are six varieties produced by Lilly, one manufacturer of insulin (Figure 8.1). Refer to a good pharmacology text for the action of the different types of insulin.

It is very important to measure insulin accurately to prevent serious problems. Insulin shock, coma, and death could occur from an untreated overdose of insulin. If insufficient insulin is received, the patient may develop hyperglycemia leading to diabetic coma and death if left untreated. Insulin dosage could be calculated in milliliters or minims in the same manner as any other dosage problem, and may be given in a tuberculin or cc syringe if absolutely necessary (most hospitals forbid this practice, however).

● A BOLD BLACK LETTER IS USED TO IDENTIFY THE TYPES OF ILETIN:
"R" (REGULAR), "P" (PROTAMINE ZINC), "N" (NPH), "L" (LENTE®), "S" (SEMILENTE®),
AND "U" (ULTRALENTE®).

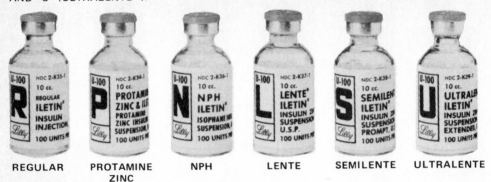

REGULAR   PROTAMINE   NPH   LENTE   SEMILENTE   ULTRALENTE
               ZINC

Figure 8.1*

*Pictures adapted from *Directions for changing from U-40 or U-80 to U-100 Iletin®* (100 units of insulin per cc), published by Eli Lilly and Company, July 1973.

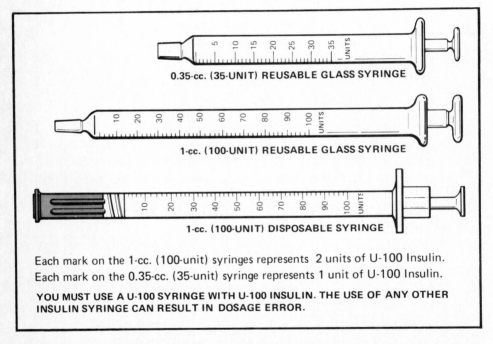

0.35-cc. (35-UNIT) REUSABLE GLASS SYRINGE

1-cc. (100-UNIT) REUSABLE GLASS SYRINGE

1-cc. (100-UNIT) DISPOSABLE SYRINGE

Each mark on the 1-cc. (100-unit) syringes represents 2 units of U-100 Insulin.
Each mark on the 0.35-cc. (35-unit) syringe represents 1 unit of U-100 Insulin.

YOU MUST USE A U-100 SYRINGE WITH U-100 INSULIN. THE USE OF ANY OTHER INSULIN SYRINGE CAN RESULT IN DOSAGE ERROR.

Figure 8.2   Three types of U-100 insulin syringes are pictured. The disposable and reusable 100 unit 1-cc syringes are used when giving larger doses of insulin. Each line represents 2 units of U-100 insulin. The 35-unit 0.35 cc syringe is for administering small doses of insulin. Each line represents 1 unit of U-100 insulin.*

*Pictures adapted from *Directions for changing from U-40 or U-80 to U-100 Iletin* ®(100 units of insulin per cc), published by Eli Lilly and Company, July 1973.

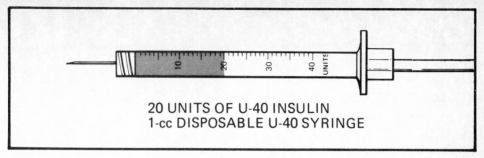

Figure 8.3

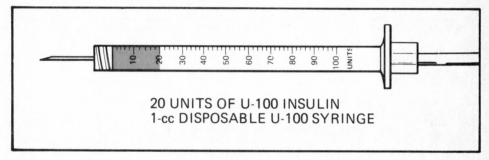

Figure 8.4

*Pictures adapted from *Directions for changing from U-40 or U-80 to U-100 Iletin* ®(100 units of insulin per cc), published by Eli Lilly and Company, July 1973.

20 units of the correct strength insulin are measured in each type of syringe. U-40 and U-100.

Draw 20 units of U-40 insulin up to the 20 unit mark on the U-40 syringe. (Figure 8.3).

Draw 20 units of U-100 insulin up to the 20 unit mark on the U-100 syringe. (Figure 8.4)

There is nothing complicated about administering insulin. Just be certain you choose the correct type of insulin and match the strength of the insulin with the syringe that matches the units per milliliter of the insulin being administered. For test purposes, you will be required to state the type of syringe you will use with the insulin ordered and what calibration you will draw the insulin to in the syringe.

1. Prepare 30 units of U-40 Regular insulin.

   Type syringe?
   Type of insulin?
   How would you prepare it?

2. Prepare 90 units of U-100 N.P.H. insulin.

 Type syringe?
 Type of insulin?
 How would you prepare it?

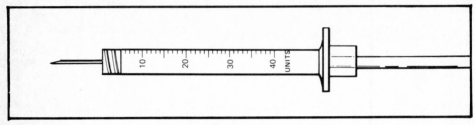

Figure 8.5

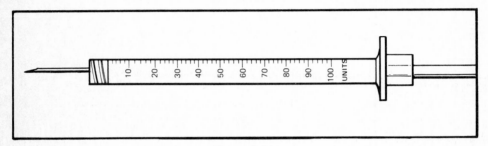

Figure 8.6

 Choose the correct syringe for each of the above problems and shade in the dosage correctly for each of the above problems.

ANSWERS TO INSULIN PROBLEMS

1. Use a U-40 insulin syringe.
 Use 40 unit/ml Regular insulin.
 Draw 40 unit/ml Regular insulin up to the 30 unit mark on a U-40 syringe.

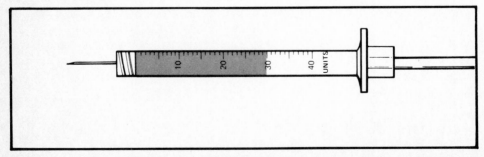

Figure 8.7

2. Use a U-100 insulin syringe.
   Use 100 unit/ml N.P.H. insulin.
   Draw 100 unit/ml N.P.H. insulin up to the 90 unit mark on a U-100 syringe.

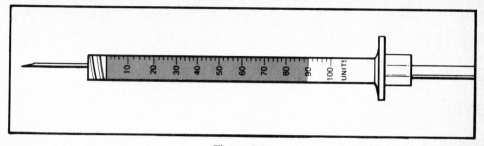

Figure 8.8

9　Reconstituting Drugs in Powdered or Crystalline Form

OBJECTIVES

After completing this chapter, the student will be able to:

1. *Select the correct diluent*
2. *State the correct amount of diluent needed to reconstitute the drug*
3. *Follow the mixing instructions stated on the bottle to prepare the solution*
4. *Find the dosage strength of the solution on the label and use it to complete the dosage problem*
5. *Define drug displacement*
6. *Identify storage instructions*
7. *Identify the stability period of the drug*
8. *Choose the correct strength to mix a drug when several choices of mixing instructions are given.*

Some drugs are unstable in liquid form. These drugs are dispensed in crystalline or powdered form. The nurse must add the diluent according to the manufacturer's instructions. After carefully following the mixing instructions, the nurse must then look for the strength of the reconstituted drug and administer the correct dosage. The usual diluents are normal saline or sterile water for injection. The drugs are dispensed in either single dose or multi-dose vials.

Look at the label. Easy to follow directions are included to prepare the solution. Simply follow the directions step by step. For example,

1. Look at the Keflin label.

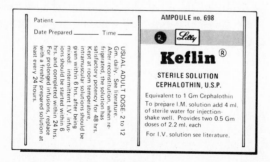

Figure 9.1*

*This label is not currently in use. Keflin is usually given IV. Used by special permission of Earl Scott Jr., Dept. Head, Printed Packaging Materials, Eli Lilly and Company.

2. Mix the drug as instructed—add 4 ml of sterile water for injection, and SHAKE WELL. Your solution is now made. You do not need to do anything more with these instructions.
3. Now look for the dosage strength of the solution of Keflin. You will see that the solution you just mixed provides two 0.5 gm doses of 2.2 ml each. Use these figures to compute your dosage.

If the doctor has ordered 0.5 gm, you must give 2.2 ml.
If the doctor has ordered 0.25 gm, you must give 1.1 ml.

$$\frac{\overset{1}{\cancel{0.25}} \text{ gm}}{\underset{2}{\cancel{0.5}} \text{ gm}} \times 2.2 \text{ ml} = 1.1 \text{ ml}$$

If the doctor has ordered 1 gm, you must give 4.4 ml.

$$\frac{\overset{2}{\cancel{1} \text{ gm}}}{\underset{1}{\cancel{0.5} \text{ gm}}} \times 2.2 \text{ ml} = 4.4 \text{ ml}$$

DISPLACEMENT

When 1 gm of Keflin was mixed with 4 ml of sterile water for injection, the resulting solution contained 2 - 0.5 gm doses of 2.2 ml each. The total solution measured 4.4 ml. The extra 0.4 ml volume resulted from the space required by the 1 gm of Keflin. The pharmaceutical company allowed for the drug displacement by adding the extra 0.4 ml of solution to the dosage strength of the drug, 1 gm of Keflin/4.4 ml. The amount of drug displacement is different for each drug.

In some instances, the hospital may not stock the dosage strength you need, but will send a unit dose vial containing a larger dose than you will give. The pharmaceutical company assumes that you are going to give the entire contents of the vial. You may only need a portion of the vial. After mixing the drug, measure the resulting solution and *calculate the dosage from the measured amount*, remembering there is drug displacement in all solutions. The larger the quantity of drug, the greater the displacement.

Example

Loridine 1 gm
Add 2.5 ml of sterile water
The finished solution measured 3.3 ml
How much displacement occurred?

```
  3.3 ml Total solution
 -2.5 ml Solution added
 ------
  0.8 ml Displacement
```

To give 0.5 gm of Loridine, how much solution will you give?

1 gm : 3.3 ml : : 0.5 gm : X ml

　　　1 X = 1.65

　　　　or

$$\frac{0.5 \text{ gm}}{1} \times 3.3 \text{ ml} = \frac{1.65}{1} = 1.65 \text{ ml}$$

Remember, if the pharmaceutical company has not told you the amount of solution in the bottle, and you are not going to give all of the solution:

1. Measure the contents of the bottle
2. Using this measurement, calculate the amount of solution containing the correct dosage (amount ordered).

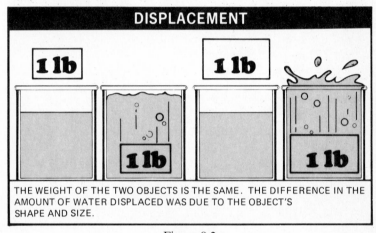

THE WEIGHT OF THE TWO OBJECTS IS THE SAME. THE DIFFERENCE IN THE AMOUNT OF WATER DISPLACED WAS DUE TO THE OBJECT'S SHAPE AND SIZE.

Figure 9.2

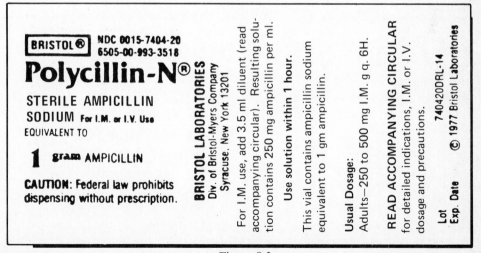

Figure 9.3

Prepare Polycillin-N® (ampicillin) (Fig. 9.3).

1. How much diluent must you add? _____

2. What is the dosage strength of this solution? _____

3. If the doctor orders 250 mg, how much solution will you give? _____

   _____

4. If the doctor orders 500 mg, how much solution will you give? _____

   _____

5. If the doctor orders 1 gm, how much solution will you give? _____

   _____

Answers

1. The amount of diluent to add is 3.5 ml.
2. The dosage strength is 250 mg per ml.
3. To give 250 mg, you would give 1 ml.
4. To give 500 mg, you would give 2 ml.

   250 mg : 1 ml : : 500 mg : X ml

   250X = 500

   X = 2 ml

5. To give 1 gm, you would give 4 ml.

   First convert 1 gm to mg = 1000 mg

   $$\frac{1000 \text{ mg}}{250 \text{ mg}} \times 1 \text{ ml} = 4 \text{ ml}$$

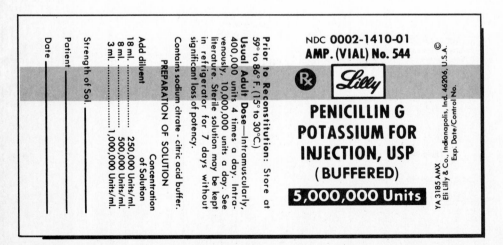

Figure 9.4

The instructions for mixing Penicillin G Potassium for injection 5,000,000 units is different. You have a choice of three different strengths for mixing this drug. Choose the dilution that will give a concentration close to the amount you must give. If the doctor orders 250,000 units for the patient, mix the Penicillin G by adding 18 ml of diluent. The resulting solution will then contain a dosage strength of 250,000 units per ml of solution. If the doctor orders 1,000,000 units of Penicillin G, you would add only 3 ml of diluent. The resulting dosage strength will be 1,000,000 units per 1 ml.

1. How much diluent must you add to the vial (ampule) if the doctor orders 500,000 units? _____

2. How much solution will you give to administer 500,000 units? _____

   _____

If the doctor orders 750,000 units to be given I M

3. How much diluent would you add? _____

4. How much solution will you administer to the patient? _____

   _____

One and a half milliliters of solution is within acceptable standards for an I M injection. The solution is not so concentrated that the injection would be irritating to the intramuscular tissue, nor so dilute that the volume of the solution would be too large. The nurse had to choose the dilution nearest to the dose ordered. Had the nurse chosen to dilute the penicillin with 3 ml of diluent the dose of penicillin would have been 0.75 ml, an acceptable amount. Had the nurse chosen to dilute the penicillin with 18 ml of the diluent, the dose to give would have been 3 ml, a larger than necessary amount that would be more painful to the patient.

Answers

1. 8 ml
2. 1 ml.   The dosage strength is 500,000 U/ml
3. Use 8 ml of diluent to make a solution of 500,000 U/ml
4. 1.5 ml

$$\frac{\overset{3}{\cancel{750,000}} \text{ U}}{\underset{2}{\cancel{500,000}} \text{ U}} \times 1 \text{ ml} \quad \frac{3}{2} = 1.5 \text{ ml of penicillin}$$

or

$$500,000 \text{ U} : 1 \text{ ml} : : 750,000 \text{ U} : X \text{ ml}$$
$$500,000 \text{ X} = 750,000$$
$$X = \frac{750,000}{500,000} = \frac{3}{2} = 1.5 \text{ ml}$$

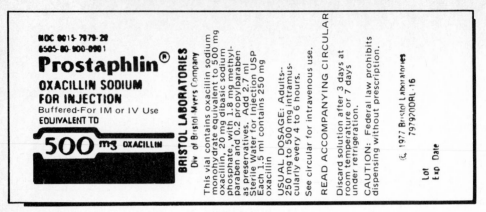

Figure 9.5

1. The doctor orders sodium oxacillin 250 mg I M

   a. How much diluent must you add? _____

   b. What diluent will you use? _____

   c. After mixing, how many days is the solution stable? _____

   d. How many ml will you give? _____

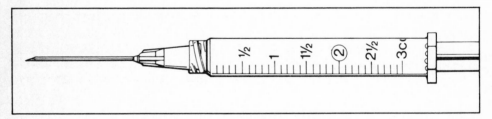

Figure 9.6   Shade syringe to proper dose.

2. The doctor orders Prostaphlin® 500 mg.

   a. How much solution will you give? _____

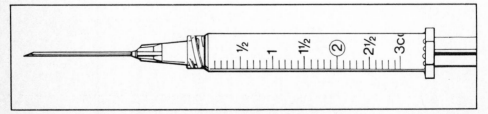

Figure 9.7   Shade syringe to proper dose.

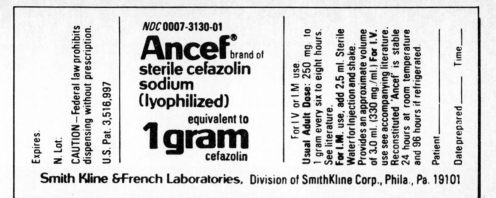

Figure 9.8

3. Prepare Ancef 1 gram for I M injection.

a. How much diluent will you use? _____

b. What diluent will you use? _____

c. How long is this reconstituted solution stable? _____

d. Administer 660 mg. How many ml will you give? _____

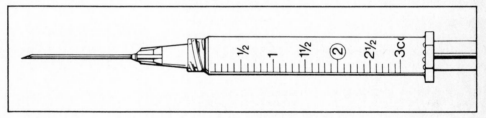

Figure 9.9   Shade syringe to correct line.

e. To administer 1 gm, how much will you give? _____

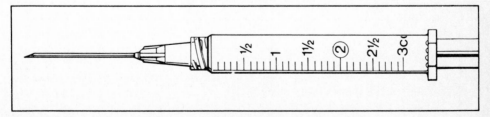

Figure 9.10   Shade syringe to correct line.

4. Prepare 1 gram of cefazolin sodium for IV administration.

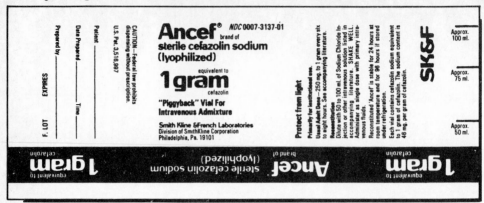

Figure 9.11   Current Ancef 1 gram for "Piggyback" vial for intravenous.

a. How much diluent must you add? _____
b. What diluent can be used? _____
c. How long is this solution stable? _____

5. Prepare 1 gram of Cefadyl for IV administration.

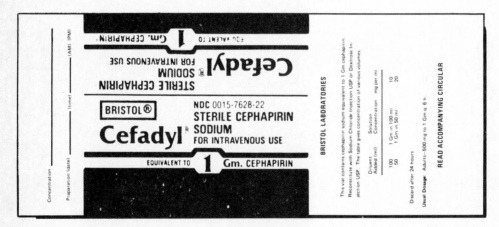

Figure 9.12

a. How much diluent must you add?   _____
b. What diluent can you use? _____
c. What special instructions are given?   _____
d. What is the usual dosage? _____
e. What is the dosage strength of each of the solutions you may prepare?
_____

ANSWERS: MIXING POWDERED DRUGS

1. a. 2.7 ml
   b. Sterile water for injection U.S.P.
   c. Discard solution after 3 days at room temperature or 7 days under refrigeration.
   d. 1.5 ml.

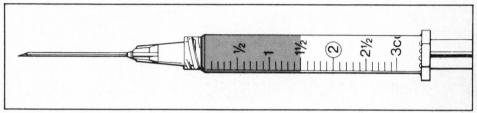

Figure 9.13

2. a. 3 ml

$$250 \text{ mg} : 1.5 \text{ ml} : : 500 \text{ mg} : X \text{ ml}$$
$$250 X = 750$$
$$X = 3 \text{ ml}$$

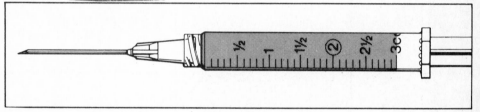

Figure 9.14

3. a. 2.5 ml
   b. Sterile water for injection.
   c. Stable for 24 hours at room temperature, 96 hours if stored under refrigeration.
   d. 2 ml

$$\frac{\overset{2}{\cancel{660}}}{\underset{1}{\cancel{330}}} \times 1 \text{ ml} = 2 \text{ ml}$$

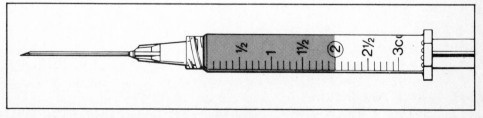

Figure 9.15

e. All of the solution, approximately 3 ml

$$330 \text{ mg} : 1 \text{ ml} : : 1000 \text{ mg} : X \text{ ml}$$
$$330 \text{ X} = 1000$$
$$X = 3 \text{ ml}$$

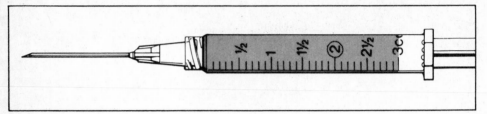

Figure 9.16

4. a. 50 to 100 ml
    b. Sodium chloride for injection or other intravenous solution listed in accompanying literature.
    c. 24 hours at room temperature, 96 hours if refrigerated.

5. a. Either 50 ml or 100 ml
    b. Sodium chloride for injection U.S.P. or dextrose injection U.S.P.
    c. Discard after 24 hours
    d. 500 mg to 1 gm q 6 h
    e. 1 gm in 100 ml, 10 gm/ml
        1 gm in 50 ml, 20 gm/ml

To mix Cefadyl you are given a choice of two strengths.

10 How to Prepare a Dosage From a Percent Solution

OBJECTIVES

After studying the content of this chapter, the student will be able to:

1. Define the meaning of percent
2. Determine the amount of solution needed to give X grams of drug from a percent solution, using either a formula or a proportion.

Remember these important points: Percent means there are X number of parts in every 100 parts. Percentage means hundredths. A percent (%) is the same as a fraction in which the denominator is 100; the numerator indicates the part of 100 being considered. For example, a 50% solution is written as a fraction, 50/100. The 50 represents the amount of drug in the solution and 100 the total solution. It is always a ratio of grams of drug to milliliters of solution. The 50 represents the number of grams of drug being considered. The 100 represents the number of milliliters of solution containing 50 gm of drug.

"The gram is the weight of 1 milliliter of distilled water at 4°C." (Bergersen, Betty S., *Pharmacology in Nursing,* 14th Edition. C. V. Mosby Co., St. Louis 1979, p. 47.) In other words, a gram and a milliliter are equivalent. This is the rationale for comparing grams of drug to milliliters of solution in a percentage solution.

To determine the amount of solution which contains X number of grams, set up a ratio and proportion.

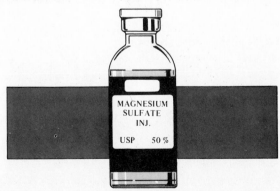

Figure 10.1

Problem:

Give 10 gms of $MgSo_4$ from a 50%* solution

$$\frac{*50\ gm}{100\ ml} :: \frac{10\ gm}{X\ ml}\ \ or\ \ 50\ gm : 100\ ml :: 10\ gm : X\ ml$$

$50\ X = 1000$

$\quad X = 20$ ml of solution

We can also use the formula $\frac{D}{H} \times V = G$

$$\frac{Dose}{strength}\ \frac{10\ gm}{50\ gm} \times 100\ ml = \frac{1000}{50} = 20\ ml\ of\ solution\ will$$
$\text{(a 50\%}$ $\qquad\qquad\qquad\qquad\qquad\qquad\qquad$ contain 10 gms of $MgSO_4$
solution)

Remember: 50% means there is 50 gm of drug in 100 ml of solution.

PROBLEMS: DOSAGE FROM A PERCENT SOLUTION

Work the following problems.

1. Prepare 2 gm of chloral hydrate from a 25% solution.

2. Give 6 gm of $MgSO_4$ from a 15% solution.

3. Give 40 gm of drug from a 70% solution.

4. Give 25 gm of drug from a 30% solution.

ANSWER: DOSAGE FROM A PERCENT SOLUTION

1. $\frac{25\ gm}{100\ ml} :: \frac{2\ gm}{X\ ml}$ $\qquad$ $\frac{2\ gm}{25\ gm} \times 100\ ml = \frac{200}{25} = 8$ ml of chloral hydrate sol

$\quad 25\ X = 200$

$\qquad X = 8$ ml of chloral hydrate sol.

2. $\dfrac{15 \text{ gm}}{100 \text{ ml}} :: \dfrac{6 \text{ gm}}{X \text{ ml}}$

    $15 \text{ X} = 600$
       $X = 40 \text{ ml MgSO}_4$

3. $70 \text{ gm} : 100 \text{ ml} :: 40 \text{ gm} : X \text{ ml}$
        $70 \text{ X} = 4000$
          $X = 57.1 \text{ or } 57 \text{ ml drug}$

4. $\dfrac{30 \text{ gm}}{100 \text{ ml}} :: \dfrac{25 \text{ gm}}{X \text{ ml}}$

    $30 \text{ X} = 2500$
       $X = 83 \ 1/3 \text{ ml or } 83 \text{ ml drug}$

$\dfrac{6 \text{ gm}}{15 \text{ gm}} \times 100 \text{ ml} = \dfrac{600}{15}$

$X = 40 \text{ ml of MgSO}_4 \text{ sol}$

$\dfrac{40 \text{ gm}}{70 \text{ gm}} \times 100 \text{ ml} = \dfrac{4000}{70}$
$= 57.1 \text{ or } 57 \text{ ml of drug}$

$\dfrac{25 \text{ gm}}{30 \text{ gm}} \times 100 \text{ ml} = \dfrac{2500}{30}$
$= 83\tfrac{1}{3} \text{ ml or } 83 \text{ ml of drug}$

11   Preparation of Solutions

OBJECTIVES

After studying the content of this chapter, the student will be able to:

1. *Define solute, solvent, diluent, solution, percent solution, and ratio strength solution*
2. *Calculate the amount of drug necessary to prepare a percent solution from a solid 100% drug*
3. *Calculate the amount of drug necessary to prepare a percent solution from a 100% liquid drug*
4. *Calculate the amount of drug necessary to prepare a ratio strength solution from a solid drug*
5. *Calculate the amount of drug necessary to prepare a ratio strength solution from a liquid drug*
6. *Calculate the amount of a stronger solution necessary to prepare a weaker solution*
7. *Calculate the amount of a solvent necessary to prepare any of the above solutions*
8. *Determine the strength of a solution, given the amount of drug dissolved in a specific amount of solution*
9. *Determine the amount of a given strength solution that may be prepared from a specified amount of drug*
10. *Determine the amount of a given strength solution that may be prepared from a specified amount of a stronger solution*
11. *Determine the percentage strength of a solution, given the amount of solute and the amount of solution.*

Nurses are occasionally required to prepare a solution for an irrigation or a soak. The pharmacist usually prepares the solution but the nurse must know how in case it is necessary. The nurse may need to teach a patient to prepare a solution for home use. It is not difficult and the formulas are very similar to the formulas for dosage.

You will need to know the medical definitions of several terms used in solution preparation.

solute: amount of drug or a chemical dissolved in a solution
solvent: liquid used to dissolve or dilute a drug or chemical to make a solution

diluent: liquid used to dissolve or dilute a drug or chemical to make a solution

solution: the liquid resulting from dissolving a solute in a diluent or a solvent

To work solution problems you may use a formula or ratio and proportion similar to those used for dosage problems. Set up the ratio and proportion.

				Desired amt.
strength desired	:	strength available	: : amt. of solute needed :	of solution
(weaker strength)		(stronger strength)	(Drug)	(Solution)

The drug, amount of solute, is usually the unknown; however, you may determine any of the other numbers in the ratio and proportion as long as you know three amounts. Think what each number represents; then fill it into the appropriate place. The strength desired and the strength available may be either a percentage strength or a ratio strength, or set up the formula:

$$\frac{\text{Strength desired}}{\text{Strength available}} \quad \frac{D}{H} \times \text{Desired amount of Solution} = \text{Amount of Solute needed}$$

PERCENTAGE SOLUTIONS

Solutions may be made from pure drugs (100% drugs) in solid or liquid form. Examples of pure drugs in crystalline or powdered form are sodium chloride, boric acid, and magnesium sulfate. Examples of pure liquid drugs include glycerin and cresol. Remember, percent is the amount of drug (grams if solid, milliliters if liquid) dissolved in 100 ml of solution.

Using a Liquid Drug

Prepare 1000 ml of a 40% lysol solution. Pure lysol is considered a 100% liquid drug so we will use the ratio 40 ml : 100 ml.

METHOD I

Step 1: Set up a ratio and proportion.

% Desired : Available :: Amount of solute needed : Desired amount of solution

40 ml : 100 ml :: X ml : 1000 ml
100 X = 40,000
X = 400 ml of lysol needed to prepare 1000 ml of a 40% solution

Step 2: How much solvent is needed to prepare 1000 ml of solution?

1000 ml Amount of solution desired
− 400 ml Amount of lysol needed to make 1000 ml of a 40% lysol solution
600 ml Amount of water needed to prepare the solution

METHOD II

Formula: $\dfrac{D}{H} \times$ Desired amount of solution $=$ Amount of solute needed to prepare the solution

$\dfrac{\text{\% Desired 40\% solution}}{\text{Have available 100\% solution}} \dfrac{40 \text{ ml}}{\cancel{100} \text{ ml}} \times \cancel{1000} \text{ ml} = 400 \text{ ml of lysol}$

$\qquad\qquad\qquad\qquad\qquad\qquad 1$

Finish problem as in Step 2 above.

CAUTION: When you are preparing solutions, your formula looks similar to a dosage problem and is worked the same way, but you are not looking for the amount to administer in your answer. You are looking for the *amount of drug or solute* to be dissolved in a solvent to make a solution. Your answer will be in grams of drug (or milliliters of drug, if the solute is a liquid, as in the first example where you used a 100% lysol solution). In the dosage problems, you have been finding *the number of tablets* or *the amount of solution* containing the desired drug dosage.

Using a Solid Drug (tablets, crystal, or powder)

Prepare 250 ml. of a 0.9%* solution of salt for a gargle.

Step 1: Use the ratio and proportion

% strength desired		% strength available		Amount of solute needed		Desired amount of solution
0.9 gm	:	100 ml	::	X gm	:	250 ml

$100X = 225$

$\qquad X = 2.25$ gm of salt

OR

Use the formula for this problem if you desire.

$\dfrac{D}{H} \times V \text{ (desired volume)} = \text{Solute}$

$\dfrac{0.9 \text{ gm}}{100 \text{ ml}} \times 250 \text{ ml} = 2.25 \text{ gm of salt}$

Step 2: If salt crystals are to be used, weigh 2.25 gm of salt. Add it to a measuring graduate and add sufficient water to make 250 ml. Remember a solid drug will take up space in the solution (displacement). You do not know how much space it will take. Always add the solid drug to the mixing container first, then add sufficient solvent to make the desired amount of solution. Tablets of known strength may be used to prepare solutions.

Alternate Step 2: If the preparation to be used is in tablet form instead of crystals, you may need to set up a dosage problem to find out how many tablets to dissolve to make the solution.

Use 1 gm salt tablets to make the gargle.

1 gm : 1 tab. :: 2.25 gm : X tab. $\qquad$ OR $\qquad \dfrac{2.25 \text{ gm}}{1 \text{ gm}} \times 1 \text{ tab.} = 2\frac{1}{4} \text{ tab.}$

$\qquad 1 X = 2.25 \text{ or } 2\frac{1}{4} \text{ tablets}$

*A 0.9% salt or saline solution is considered physiologic saline. It is isotonic with body fluids.

Dissolve 2¼ tablets in a small amount of water then add sufficient water to make 250 ml of saline gargle.

If you are to instruct a patient how to prepare a saline gargle at home, you could instruct the patient to dissolve ½ teaspoon of salt in an 8 oz glass of warm water and gargle X number of times a day as ordered by the doctor.

Remember, 1 teaspoon = 4 to 5 ml
2.25 gm = approximately ½ teaspoon

This is permissible for a gargle but drugs to be taken internally should *NEVER* be approximated.

Preparation of a Weaker Solution from a Stronger Solution

Weaker solutions may be made from stronger solutions. Examples of solutions that may be kept as stock drugs in concentrated form are potassium permanganate and benzalkonium chloride. The strength of these solutions may be expressed as a percentage strength or as a ratio strength. Set up the first ratio weaker drug to stronger drug. To prepare a weaker solution from a stronger solution set up the following ratio:

Strength : Strength   Amount of   Amount of
 desired : available ::   solute   :   solution
(weaker) : (stronger)   to use   desired

Prepare 2000 ml of a 6% cresol solution from a 10% solution of cresol.

Step 1: D   : H   :: solute : solution
       6% : 10% :: X ml : 2000 ml
       6 ml : 10 ml :: X ml : 2000 ml
           10 X = 12000
              X = 1200 ml   Use 1200 ml of the 10% cresol solution to make
                            2000 ml of a 6% cresol solution.

Step 2: Find the amount of solvent to be used.
        2000   amount of solution
      − 1200   amount of solute
         800   ml of water needs to be added to the 1200 ml of 10% cresol to
               make a 6% cresol solution.

Formula: $\dfrac{D}{H} \times$ Amt. of solution = Amt. of solute

Step 1: $\dfrac{6\%}{10\%} \times 2000 =$

$\dfrac{6 \text{ ml}}{10 \text{ ml}} \times 2000 \text{ ml} = \dfrac{12000}{10} = 1200 \text{ ml of } 10\% \text{ Cresol}$

Step 2: Same as above

Preparation of a Ratio Strength Solution

Prepare 500 ml of $KMnO_4$ 1:10000 solution from a 1:5000 solution of $KMnO_4$. This may be worked as fractions or it may be changed to percents.

$$D \quad : \quad H \quad :: \quad \text{Solute} : \text{Solution}$$

Step 1: $\dfrac{1}{10000} : \dfrac{1}{5000} :: X \text{ ml sol} : 500 \text{ ml}$

$$\frac{1}{5000} X = \frac{500}{10000}$$

$$\frac{1}{5000} \div \frac{1}{5000} X = \frac{500}{10000} \div \frac{1}{5000}$$

$$\frac{\cancel{1}}{\cancel{5000}} \times \frac{\cancel{5000}}{\cancel{1}} X = \frac{500}{\underset{2}{\cancel{10000}}} \times \frac{\overset{1}{\cancel{5000}}}{1}$$

$$X = \frac{500}{2}$$

$X = 250$ ml. Use 250 ml of the 1:5000 solution of $KMnO_4$ to make 500 ml of a 1:10000 solution of $KMnO_4$.

Done as a percent. (Ratio strengths may be changed to percent.)

$0.01\% : 0.02\% :: X \text{ ml} : 500 \text{ ml}$

$0.02 X = 5$

$$X = \frac{5}{.02}$$

$X = 250$ ml of solute 1:5000 $KMnO_4$

Step 2:
    500 ml   solution desired
   − 250 ml   amount of solute
    250 ml   of water needed

OR

Formula: $\dfrac{D}{H} \times V = \text{Solute}$

$$\frac{\dfrac{1}{10000 \text{ ml}}}{\dfrac{1}{5000 \text{ ml}}} \times \frac{500 \text{ ml}}{1} = \frac{\dfrac{500}{10000}}{\dfrac{1}{5000}}$$

$$\frac{500}{10000} \div \frac{1}{5000} = \frac{500}{\underset{2}{\cancel{10000}}} \times \frac{\overset{1}{\cancel{5000}}}{1} = \frac{500}{2} = 250 \text{ ml of the } 1:5000$$
solution of $KMnO_4$

Work Step 2 as above.

Preparation of an Unknown Quantity of Solution When the Amount of Solute (Drug) Is Known

Set up this type of problem using the same proportion used for other solution problems. The only difference in this problem and the other problems is that the quantity of solution is the unknown factor, the amount of solute is known.

Using 90 ml of lysol, prepare a 5% solution. How much solution can be made?

Desired strength	:	Available strength	::	Amount of solute	:	Amount of solution
5%	:	100%	::	90 ml	:	X ml
5 ml	:	100 ml	::	90 ml	:	X ml

$$5X = 9000$$
$$X = 1800 \text{ ml of a 5\% solution can be made from } 90 \text{ ml of } 100\% \text{ lysol}$$

Formula:

$$\frac{D}{H} \times X = \text{Amount of solute}$$

$$\frac{5 \text{ ml}}{100 \text{ ml}} \times X \text{ ml} = 90 \text{ ml}$$

$$\frac{5}{100} \div \frac{5}{100} X = 90 \div \frac{5}{100}$$

$$\frac{\cancel{5}}{\cancel{100}} \times \frac{\cancel{100}}{\cancel{5}} X = 90 \times \frac{\overset{20}{\cancel{100}}}{\underset{1}{\cancel{5}}}$$

$$X = 1800 \text{ ml of 5\% solution}$$

Proof
$$\frac{5 \text{ ml}}{100 \text{ ml}} \times 1800 \text{ ml} = \frac{9000}{100} = 90 \text{ ml}$$

Determining the Percent of a Solution

Nurses frequently state that they do not need to know how to prepare solutions. The pharmacist does it for them. A nursing drug paper presented a story, reprinted from JAMA, about a baby brought into the hospital unable to breathe because the mucous membranes of her nose were swollen, cutting off her breath, causing acute nasal obstruction and respiratory distress. The mother had been instructed to make saline nose drops to use in the baby's nose. When the mother was questioned, it was found she had prepared the nose drops by using 1 tablespoon of salt to 8 oz of water.*

*Ulin, I.S., Bartlett G.: Iatrogenic acute nasal obstruction in an obligate nose breather. JAMA 243: 1657 (April 25) 1980.

To determine the percent of the solution prepared by the mother, set up a proportion using the known quantities. The mother added 1 tablespoon of salt to an 8 ounce glass of warm water.

Known Facts: 1 Tablespoon = 15 ml

1 gm of a drug is equal to 1 ml of water at 4°C

A percent is the number of grams of drug in 100 ml of solution.

8 oz = 240 ml

From these facts set up a proportion:

$$\frac{X \text{ gm}}{100 \text{ ml}} :: \frac{15 \text{ gm}}{240 \text{ ml}}$$

$$240 \text{ X} = 1500$$
$$X = 6.25 \text{ gm}$$

Place the value of X over 100 and change to a percent

$$\frac{6.25 \text{ gm}}{100 \text{ ml}} = 0.0625 = 6.25\% \text{ solution was prepared by the mother}$$

The mother had prepared a 6.25% solution. The mother should have prepared a 0.5% solution by using ¼ teaspoon of salt to an eight ounce glass of water. Regardless of why this mother prepared the wrong strength solution, nurses are frequently the ones who are responsible for teaching patients/clients how to prepare similar kinds of solutions. It is of the utmost importance that nurses be able to instruct others correctly and/or be able to prepare a solution in the correct strength. Nurses may not prepare solutions frequently, but they should be able to prepare them correctly when necessary.

PROBLEMS: SOLUTION PREPARATION

1. Prepare 1000 ml of physiologic saline 0.9% using 1 gm salt tablets.

2. Prepare 500 ml of a 10% solution of a boric acid solution from crystals.

3. Using 1 ounce of a 2% hydrogen peroxide solution prepare a 1% solution. How much solution will this make?

4. Prepare 1 liter of 1:1000 potassium permanganate solution from a 1:500 potassium permanganate solution.

5. You are told to give 10 ml of a 10% solution. If you give this amount, how do you know it is equal to 1 gm of drug—the amount ordered by the doctor?

6. Prepare 1 pint of a 2% solution from 250 mg tablets.

7. Prepare a 5% solution using 30 ml of drug.

8. Prepare 400 ml of a ½% solution from a 5% solution.

9. Prepare 2 gallons of a 15% solution of lysol from pure lysol.

10. Prepare 800 ml of a 25% solution of $MgSO_4$ solution from $MgSO_4$ crystals.

11. How much 10% solution would be needed to make 1 gallon of a 3% solution? How much water would be needed?

12. How much of a 5% solution would be needed to prepare 1500 ml of a 2% solution? How much water would be needed?

13. How much of a 1:5 stock solution would be needed to prepare 1 liter of a 1:20 solution? How much water would be needed?

14. How much of a 1:2000 solution would be needed to prepare 4000 ml of a 1:10,000 solution? How much water would be needed?

15. How much vinegar is necessary to make 1000 ml of a 4% solution? How much water would be needed?

16. If 30 gm of drug was used to prepare 1000 ml of solution, what is the percentage strength of this solution?

17. If 250 ml of glycerine was used to prepare 4000 ml of solution, what is the percentage strength of this solution?

ANSWERS: SOLUTION PREPARATION

1. *Step 1:* 0.9 gm : 100 ml :: X gm : 1000 ml
$$100 X = 900$$
$$X = 9 \text{ gm of salt}$$

Step 2: 1 gm : 1 tab. :: 9 gm : X tab
$$1 X = 9 \text{ tablets of salt}$$

Dissolve 9 tablets of salt in enough water to make 1000 ml of solution.

2. $\dfrac{10 \text{ gm}}{\underset{1}{100 \text{ ml}}} \times \overset{5}{500} \text{ ml} = 50 \text{ gm}$

Weigh 50 gm of boric acid crystals and dissolve in enough water to make 500 ml

3. D : H :: Solute : Solution   1 oz = 30 ml

1% : 2% :: 30 ml : X ml
$$1 X = 60 \text{ ml of solution of } H_2O_2 \text{ can be made}$$

In this problem, you have 30 ml of a 2% solution. You had to find out how much 1% solution this would make.

4. 1 L = 1000 ml. Remember values must be in the same unit of measure. You must convert liters to milliliters.

$$\frac{\dfrac{1}{1000}}{\dfrac{1}{500}} \times 1000 \text{ ml} = \frac{\dfrac{1000}{1000}}{\dfrac{1}{500}} = \frac{1000}{1000} \div \frac{1}{500}$$

$$= \frac{\overset{1}{\cancel{1000}}}{\underset{1}{\cancel{1000}}} \times \frac{500}{1} = 500 \text{ ml KMnO}_4$$

5. Set up a ratio and proportion to check it.

   10 gm : 100 ml :: X gm : 10 ml

   100 X = 100

   X = 1 gm

You would be right giving 10 ml.

Remember, a ratio and proportion may be used to find any part of the proportion if you know the other three values.

6. 1 pt = 500 ml

   Step 1: $\dfrac{2 \text{ gm}}{\underset{1}{\cancel{100}} \text{ ml}} \times \overset{5}{\cancel{500}} \text{ ml} = 10 \text{ gm of drug} \qquad 10 \text{ gm} = 10000 \text{ mg}$

   Step 2: Set up a dosage problem to find out how many 250 mg tablets are needed.

   $$\frac{10000 \text{ mg}}{250 \text{ mg}} \times 1 \text{ tab.} = 40 \text{ tablets}$$

   Dissolve 40 tablets of drug in sufficient water to make 1 pint of solution.

7. $\dfrac{5 \text{ ml}}{100 \text{ ml}} \times V = 30 \text{ ml} \qquad \text{OR} \qquad 5 \text{ ml} : 100 \text{ ml} :: 30 \text{ ml} : X \text{ ml}$

   $\dfrac{5}{100} \div \dfrac{5}{100} V = 30 \div \dfrac{5}{100} \qquad\qquad 5 X = 3000$

   $\qquad\qquad\qquad\qquad\qquad\qquad\qquad\qquad X = 600 \text{ ml of solution}$

   $\dfrac{\cancel{5}}{\cancel{100}} \times \dfrac{\cancel{100}}{\cancel{5}} V = 30 \times \dfrac{100}{5}$

   $V = \overset{6}{\cancel{30}} \times \dfrac{100}{\cancel{5}}$

   $V = 600 \text{ ml of solution can be made.}$

8. *Step 1:* $\dfrac{0.5}{5} :: \dfrac{\text{X ml}}{400 \text{ ml}}$

$1/2\% = 2\overline{)1.0}^{\,.5}$

$5\text{ X} = 200.0$

$\text{X} = 40 \text{ ml of drug}$

Step 2: 400 ml amount of solution desired

$\underline{\quad 40 \text{ ml}}$ of drug needed

360 ml water needed to make 400 ml of solution

9. *Step 1:* $\dfrac{15}{\cancel{100}} \times \overset{80}{\cancel{8000}} \text{ ml} = 1200 \text{ ml of pure lysol}$ $\quad$ 2 gal = 8000 ml

Step 2: 8000 ml of lysol solution desired

$\underline{-1200}$ ml pure lysol

6800 ml water needed to prepare the solution

10. *Step 1:* $\dfrac{25 \text{ gm}}{100 \text{ ml}} :: \dfrac{\text{X gm}}{800 \text{ ml}}$

$100 \text{ X} = 20000$

$\text{X} = 200 \text{ gm}$

Step 2: Add 200 gm of $MgSO_4$ crystals to a measuring graduate and add sufficient water to make 800 ml

11. How much 10% solution would be needed to make 1 gallon of a 3% solution? How much water would be needed?

$\quad$ 3 ml : 10 ml :: X ml : 4000 ml $\qquad$ 4000 ml solution desired

$\qquad\qquad$ 10 X = 12000 $\qquad\qquad\quad$ $\underline{1200}$ ml of 10% solution

$\qquad\qquad\quad$ X = 1200 ml $\qquad\qquad$ 2800 ml of water needed

$\qquad\qquad\qquad$ OR

$\qquad \dfrac{3 \text{ ml}}{10 \text{ ml}} \times \overset{400}{\cancel{4000}} \text{ ml} = 1200 \text{ ml}$

12. How much of a 5% solution would be needed to prepare 1500 ml of a 2% solution? How much water would be needed?

$\quad$ 2 ml : 5 ml :: X ml : 1500 ml $\qquad$ 1500 ml solution desired

$\qquad\qquad$ 5 X = 3000 $\qquad\qquad\qquad$ $\underline{\ 600}$ ml of 5% solution

$\qquad\qquad\quad$ X = 600 ml of 5% solution $\quad$ 900 ml H_2O needed

$\qquad\qquad\qquad$ OR

$\qquad \dfrac{2 \text{ ml}}{\cancel{5} \text{ ml}} \times \overset{300}{\cancel{1500}} \text{ ml} = 600 \text{ ml of 5\% solution}$

13. How much of a 1:5 stock solution would be needed to prepare 1 liter of a 1:20 solution? How much water would be needed?

1:20 : 1:5 :: X ml : 1000 ml   1000 ml solution needed
5 ml : 20 ml :: X ml : 1000 ml $\underline{-250}$ ml of 1:5 solution
      20 X = 5000   750 ml of water needed
           X = 250 ml

OR

$$\dfrac{\frac{1}{20}}{\frac{1}{5}} \times 1000 = \dfrac{\frac{1000}{20}}{\frac{1}{5}} = \dfrac{1000}{\cancel{20}_{4}} \times \dfrac{\cancel{5}^{1}}{1} = \dfrac{1000}{4} = 250\ ml$$

14. How much of a 1:2000 solution would be needed to prepare 4000 ml of a 1:10,000 solution? How much water would be needed?

1:10,000 : 1:2000 : X ml : 4000 ml   4000 ml solution needed
                             $\underline{800}$ ml of 1:2000 solution
$$\dfrac{1}{2000}\,X = \dfrac{4000}{10000}$$
                             3200 ml of H_2O needed

$$\dfrac{1}{2000} \div \dfrac{1}{2000}\,X = \dfrac{4000}{10000} \div \dfrac{1}{2000}$$

$$\dfrac{\cancel{1}}{\cancel{2000}} \times \dfrac{\cancel{2000}}{1}\,X = \dfrac{\overset{800}{\cancel{4000}}}{\underset{5}{\cancel{10000}}} \times \dfrac{\cancel{2000}}{1}\,X = 800\ ml\ of\ 1:2000\ solution$$

OR

$$\dfrac{\frac{1}{10000}}{\frac{1}{2000}} \times 4000 = \dfrac{\frac{4000}{10000}}{\frac{1}{2000}} = \dfrac{\overset{800}{\cancel{4000}}}{\underset{5}{\cancel{10000}}} \times \dfrac{\cancel{2000}}{1} = 800\ ml\ of\ 1:2000\ solution$$

15. How much vinegar is necessary to make 1000 ml of a 4% solution? How much water would be needed?

4 ml : 100 ml :: X ml : 1000 ml   1000 ml solution needed
      100 X = 4000 $\underline{40}$ ml vinegar
            X = 40 ml of vinegar   960 ml H_2O needed

OR

$$\dfrac{4\ ml}{\cancel{100}\ ml} \times \overset{10}{\cancel{1000}}\ ml = 40\ ml\ of\ vinegar$$

16. If 30 gm of drug was used to prepare 1000 ml of solution, what is the percentage strength of this solution?

$$\frac{X \text{ gm}}{100 \text{ ml}} :: \frac{30 \text{ gm}}{1000 \text{ ml}}$$

$1000X = 3000$

$X = 3$ gm of drug /100 ml

$\frac{3 \text{ gm}}{100 \text{ ml}} = 100 \overset{.03}{\overline{)3.00}} = 3\%$ solution

17. If 250 ml of glycerine was used to prepare 4000 ml of solution, what is the percentage strength of this solution?

$$\frac{X \text{ ml}}{100 \text{ ml}} :: \frac{250 \text{ ml}}{4000 \text{ ml}}$$

$4000X = 25,000$

$X = 6.25$ ml

$\frac{6.25 \text{ ml}}{100 \text{ ml}} = 100 \overset{0.0625}{\overline{)6.2500}} = 6.25\%$ solution

12 Intravenous Fluid Rate Calculation

OBJECTIVES

After completion of this chapter, the student will be able to:

1. *Calculate the one-hour volume from a twenty-four-hour volume of IV fluid*
2. *Use the formula given to calculate the number of drops per minute needed to administer a given volume of intravenous fluid. Use an administration set with a drop factor of 10, 15, 20 or 60 gtts/ml.*
3. *Calculate the flow rate of an IV administration set using a drop factor other than 10, 15, 20, or 60.*
4. *Calculate the flow rate of IV medications to be administered in small volumes of intravenous fluid.*
5. *Calculate the volume of intravenous fluid containing a specified amount of drug to be administered in an hour.*

Nurses frequently have to start and monitor IV solutions. It is very important to monitor IV solutions carefully because of the inherent dangers of parenteral administration. The flow rate of intravenous fluids is controlled by calibrated administration sets which administer 10, 15, 20, or 60 drops (gtts)/ml. This rate is termed the drop factor. A few IV sets used to administer special IV preparations may have a different drop factor, but these are the rates most frequently used. The physician may order IV fluids to run for a given period of time. The nurse must first calculate the one hour volume, then the drops/minute must be calculated. The formulas given here are very easy. Once you understand them there is a shortcut given that may be calculated in your head. Memorize this formula—you will use it frequently.

Formula: $\dfrac{\text{Drop factor}}{60 \text{ min in 1 hr}} \times \dfrac{\text{Total 1 hr}}{\text{volume}} = \dfrac{\text{drops per minute to be}}{\text{administered via IV set}}$

Example: Give 1000 cc of 5% Dextrose in water. IV is to run 8 hrs. Administration set runs at 10 gtts/ml (drop factor).
The nurse must know the total volume to be given and the rate of the set.

Step 1   First divide the number of hours the IV is to run (8 hrs) into the total amount of IV fluid (1000 cc) to obtain the total 1 hr volume.

$$\frac{125 \text{ cc} = 1 \text{ hr volume}}{8 \text{ hr}\ )\ 1000 \text{ cc} = 8 \text{ hr volume}}$$

Step 2   Set up the formula, substituting numbers.

$$\frac{\text{(Drop factor)}}{\underset{60 \text{ min in 1 hr}}{\text{Drops per ml of set}}} \times \underset{\text{volume}}{\text{Total 1 hr}} = \underset{\text{be administered}}{\text{drops per minute to}}$$

$$\frac{10 \text{ gtts/ml}}{60 \text{ min}} \times 125 \text{ cc} = \text{drops per minute}$$

$$\frac{\overset{1}{\cancel{10}}}{\underset{6}{\cancel{60}}} \times 125 = \frac{125}{6} = 20\ 5/6 \text{ or } 21 \text{ gtts*/min}$$

Round off to the nearest whole number.

IV CALCULATION SHORTCUT

Once you become familiar with IV flow rate calculation, you will realize that the fraction formed by placing the drop factor over 60 minutes may be reduced so that you are actually dividing the 1 hour volume by one of four numbers. If you figure out this number for the IV set used in the hospital where you are working, you only have to divide the 1 hour volume by the magic number to get the drops per minute an IV set must run to deliver the 1 hour volume.

Manufacturer	Drop Factor	Magic Number	
Abbott	Approximately 15 gtts/cc	$\dfrac{15}{60}$	4
Baxter	" 10 gtts/cc	$\dfrac{10}{60}$	6
Cutter	" 20 gtts/cc	$\dfrac{20}{60}$	3
Any mini or micro dropper	" 60 gtts/cc	$\dfrac{60}{60}$	1

*gtt = the abbreviation for "gutta," Latin for drop.

Doctor's order: Run IV at 125 ml/hr

$$\frac{\text{Drop factor}}{60 \text{ minutes}} \times 1 \text{ hour volume} = \text{drops/minute IV is to run}$$

If we use a set that flows 15 gtts/ml

$$\frac{\overset{1}{\cancel{15}}}{\underset{4}{\cancel{60}}} \times 125 = \frac{125}{④} = 31\tfrac{1}{4} \text{ or } 31 \text{ gtts/min}$$

If we use a set that flows 10 gtts/ml

$$\frac{\overset{1}{\cancel{10}}}{\underset{6}{\cancel{60}}} \times 125 = \frac{125}{⑥} = 20 \tfrac{5}{6} \text{ or } 21 \text{ gtts/min}$$

If we use a set that flows 20 gtts/ml

$$\frac{\overset{1}{\cancel{20}}}{\underset{3}{\cancel{60}}} \times 125 = \frac{125}{③} = 41 \tfrac{2}{3} \text{ or } 42 \text{ gtts/min}$$

If we use a micro set that flows 60 gtts/ml

$$\frac{\overset{1}{\cancel{60}}}{\underset{1}{\cancel{60}}} \times 125 = \frac{125}{①} \text{ or } 125 \text{ gtts/min}$$

NOTE: In each case above, the magic number is circled.

There are some IV sets that may have a different flow rate used for administering special solutions. Use the formula to calculate the flow rate as above. Always be sure to check for the drop factor and regulate the IV accordingly.

IV Administration of Medications in Small Volume IVs

Medications are frequently administered to patients in 50 to 100 ml of intravenous fluid. The administration time may be 30 to 60 minutes. The length of time for administration and the dilution of the drug depends on the stability and/or the irritability of the particular drug. See drug guidelines or consult the pharmacist. The IV should be maintained at the correct flow rate to prevent complications.

To calculate the flow rate of small volume IVs use the same formula substituting the actual time of administration and the volume to be administered.

$$\frac{\text{gtt factor}}{\text{length of time IV is to infuse}} \times \frac{\text{Volume to}}{\text{be infused}} = \text{gtts/min} \qquad \text{IV is to infuse}$$

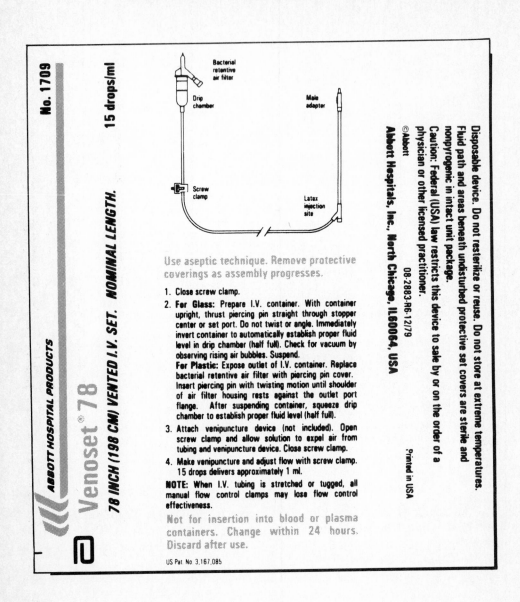

No. 1709

ABBOTT HOSPITAL PRODUCTS

Venoset® 78

78 INCH (198 CM) VENTED I.V. SET. NOMINAL LENGTH.

15 drops/ml

Bacterial
retentive
air filter

Drip
chamber

Screw
clamp

Male
adapter

Latex
injection
site

Use aseptic technique. Remove protective coverings as assembly progresses.

1. Close screw clamp.
2. **For Glass:** Prepare I.V. container. With container upright, thrust piercing pin straight through stopper center or set port. Do not twist or angle. Immediately invert container to automatically establish proper fluid level in drip chamber (half full). Check for vacuum by observing rising air bubbles. Suspend.
   For Plastic: Expose outlet of I.V. container. Replace bacterial retentive air filter with piercing pin cover. Insert piercing pin with twisting motion until shoulder of air filter housing rests against the outlet port flange. After suspending container, squeeze drip chamber to establish proper fluid level (half full).
3. Attach venipuncture device (not included). Open screw clamp and allow solution to expel air from tubing and venipuncture device. Close screw clamp.
4. Make venipuncture and adjust flow with screw clamp. 15 drops delivers approximately 1 ml.

NOTE: When I.V. tubing is stretched or tugged, all manual flow control clamps may lose flow control effectiveness.

Not for insertion into blood or plasma containers. Change within 24 hours. Discard after use.

US Pat. No. 3,167,085

Disposable device. Do not resterilize or reuse. Do not store at extreme temperatures. Fluid path and areas beneath undisturbed protective set covers are sterile and nonpyrogenic in intact unit package.

Caution: Federal (USA) law restricts this device to sale by or on the order of a physician or other licensed practitioner.

© Abbott

Abbott Hospitals, Inc., North Chicago, IL 60064, USA

08-2883-R6-12/79

Printed in USA

Figure 12.1   Drop Factor = 15 drops/ml

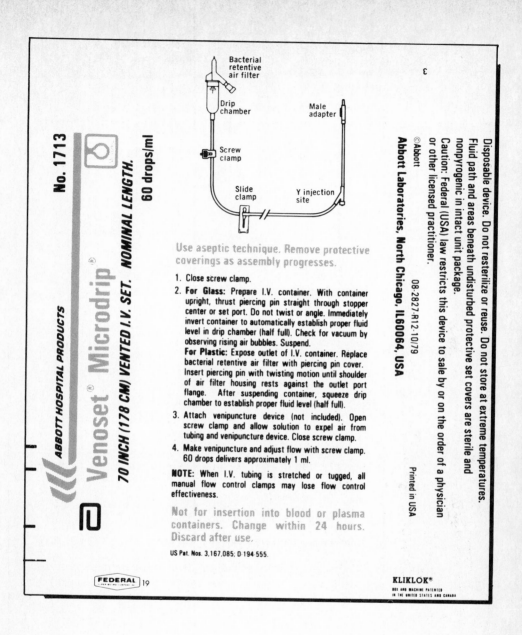

Figure 12.2   Drop Factor = 60 drops/ml

Determine the Amount of IV Fluid Containing an Ordered Amount of Drug

The doctor may order a specified amount of drug to be placed in a certain volume of intravenous fluid (500 ml - 1000 ml). Then order run at _____ gm, mEq, or units per hour.

Example: The doctors order: 1000 ml of D$_5$W with 20 mEq KCL added. Administer 2 mEq of KCL/hr.

Think of this problem as a dosage problem (See Chapter 6 on working dosage problems). The only difference is, you are working with a large volume of fluid.

METHOD I

$$\frac{\text{The dose ordered}}{\text{Strength on hand}} \times \text{Vehicle} = \text{Amount to give}$$

$$\frac{2 \text{ mEq}}{\underset{1}{\cancel{20}} \text{ mEq}} \times \overset{50}{\cancel{1000}} \text{ ml} = 100 \text{ ml to be administered per hour}$$

METHOD II

Drug   : Vehicle   : :Drug desired : Amount of vehicle to administer
20 mEq : 1000 ml   : :2 mEq   : X ml
$$20X = 2000$$
$$X = 100 \text{ ml to be administered per hour}$$

Once the volume of drug to be administered is determined, set up an IV problem using the drop factor of the IV administration set you are to use and determine the drops per minute to run the IV.

PROBLEMS: INTRAVENOUS FLUIDS

1. The doctor orders 3000 ml of IV fluids to run for 24 hrs. The administration set flow rate is 10 gtts per ml. How many gtts per minute must the nurse run this IV?

2. The doctor orders 1500 ml of IV fluid to run for 10 hrs. The administration set flow rate is 20 gtts per ml. How many gtts per minute must the nurse run this IV?

3. The doctor orders 240 ml of IV fluids for an infant, to run for 24 hrs. The IV administration set flow rate is 60 gtts per ml. How fast must the nurse run this IV?

4. The doctor orders 2500 ml of IV fluid to infuse for 24 hours. The IV administration set flow rate is 15 gtts per ml. How many gtts per minute must this IV run?

5. The doctor orders 3000 ml of IV fluids to be infused in 16 hrs. The IV administration flow rate is 10 gtts per ml. How fast must the nurse run this IV?

6. The doctor may give the 1 hr volume in his order so that the nurse may omit Step 1 and work the problem from Step 2.

    1000 ml of D5/W
    1000 ml of Ringers Lactate to follow
    1000 ml of D5/NS   0.9%
    Run at 125 cc per hr
              Dr. Supersat
    IV set runs 10 gtts/ml

7. The doctor orders sodium oxacillin 500 mg IV q4h. The sodium oxacillin has been mixed with 100 ml of solution. Administer the solution in 45 minutes. The drop factor is 10 gtt/ml. How many gtts/min must the nurse run this IV?

8. The doctor orders Mandol 2 gm IV q6h. The Mandol is to be mixed with 100 ml of diluent for administration. Administer the solution in 30 minutes. The drop factor is 15 gtt/ml. How many gtts/min must the nurse run this IV?

9. The doctor orders 1000 ml of D_5W with 10,000 units of heparin added. The patient is to receive 1000 units of heparin/hour. How many ml/hr must his IV run?

10. The doctor orders 1000 ml of D$_5$W with 20 gm of MgSO$_4$ added. The patient is to receive 1 gm/hr. How many ml/hr must this IV run? The drop factor is 60 gtt/ml. How many gtts/min must the nurse run this IV?

ANSWERS: INTRAVENOUS FLUIDS

1.
$$\frac{125 \text{ ml}}{24 \overline{)3000 \text{ ml}}} = \frac{1 \text{ hr volume}}{24 \text{ hr volume}}$$
$$\underline{24}$$
$$60$$
$$\underline{48}$$
$$120$$
$$\underline{120}$$

$$\frac{10 \text{ gtts/ml}}{60 \text{ min/hr}} \times 125 \text{ ml} = \text{gtts/min}$$

$$\frac{\overset{1}{\cancel{10}}}{\underset{6}{\cancel{60}}} \times 125 = \frac{125}{6} = 20 \ 5/6 \text{ or } 21 \text{ drops per minute}$$

2.
$$\frac{150 \text{ ml}}{10 \overline{)1500 \text{ ml}}} = \frac{1 \text{ hr volume}}{10 \text{ hr volume}}$$

$$\frac{\overset{1}{\cancel{20}} \text{ gtts/ml}}{\underset{3}{\cancel{60}} \text{ min}} \times 150 \text{ ml} = \text{gtts/min}$$

$$\frac{1}{\cancel{3}} \times \overset{50}{\cancel{150}} = 50 \text{ gtts per minute}$$

3.
$$\frac{10 \text{ ml}}{24 \overline{)240}} = \frac{1 \text{ hr volume}}{24 \text{ hr volume}}$$

$$\frac{\overset{1}{\cancel{60}} \text{ gtts/ml}}{\underset{1}{\cancel{60}} \text{ min}} \times 10 \text{ ml} = 10 \text{ gtts/min}$$

4.

$$\frac{104 \text{ ml}}{24 \overline{)2500 \text{ ml}}} = \frac{1 \text{ hr volume}}{24 \text{ hr volume}}$$

$$\begin{array}{r} \underline{24} \\ 100 \\ \underline{96} \\ 4 \end{array}$$

$$\frac{15 \text{ gtts/ml}}{60 \text{ min.}} \times 104 \,(1 \text{ hr volume}) = \text{gtts/min}$$

$$\frac{\overset{1}{\cancel{15}}}{\underset{4}{\cancel{60}}} \times 104 = \frac{104}{4} = 26 \text{ gtts/min}$$

5.

$$16 \overline{)\underset{}{\overset{187.5 \text{ ml}}{3000.0}}} = 16 \text{ hr volume}$$

$$\begin{array}{r} \underline{16} \\ 140 \\ \underline{128} \\ 120 \\ \underline{112} \\ 80 \end{array}$$

$$\frac{10 \text{ gtts/ml}}{60 \text{ min}} \times 187.5 \text{ ml } 1 \text{ hr volume} = \text{gtts/min}$$

$$\frac{\overset{1}{\cancel{10}}}{\underset{6}{\cancel{60}}} \times 187.5 = \frac{187.5}{6} = 31.2 \text{ or } 31 \text{ gtts/min}$$

OR

$$\frac{\overset{1}{\cancel{10}}}{\underset{6}{\cancel{60}}} \times 188 = \frac{188}{6} = 31 \ 1/3 \text{ or } 31 \text{ gtts/min}$$

6. $\dfrac{10 \text{ gtts/ml}}{60 \text{ min}} \times 125 = \text{gtts/min}$

$$\frac{\overset{1}{\cancel{10}}}{\underset{6}{\cancel{60}}} \times 125 = \frac{125}{6} = 20 \ 5/6 = 21 \text{ gtts/min}$$

7. $\dfrac{\text{drop factor}}{\text{time}} \times \text{Vol} \quad = \text{gtts/min}$

$\dfrac{10 \text{ gtt/ml}}{45 \text{ min}} \times 100 \text{ ml} = \dfrac{1000}{45} = 22\ 2/9 \text{ or } 22 \text{ gtts/minute}$

8. $\dfrac{\text{drop factor}}{\text{time}} \times \text{Vol} = \text{gtts/min}$

$\dfrac{\overset{1}{\cancel{15}} \text{ gtt/ml}}{\underset{\underset{1}{2}}{\cancel{30}} \text{ min}} \times \overset{50}{\cancel{100}} = 50 \text{ gtts/min}$

9. 10,000 Units : 1000 ml :: 1000 Units : Xml
$\qquad$ 10,000 X $=$ 1,000,000
$\qquad\qquad$ X $=$ 100 ml per hour the amount of IV patient is to receive

10. 20 gm : 1000 ml :: 1 gm : X ml
$\qquad$ 20 X $=$ 1000
$\qquad\qquad$ X $=$ 50 ml/hr the amount of IV patient is to receive

OR

$\dfrac{\cancel{X} \text{ gm}}{\underset{1}{\cancel{20}} \text{ gm}} \times \overset{50}{\cancel{1000}} \text{ ml} = 50 \text{ ml/hr the amount of IV patient is to receive}$

$\dfrac{60 \text{ gtt/ml}}{60 \text{ min}} \times 50 \text{ ml} = 50 \text{ gtts/min} = \text{IV flow rate}$

13   Pediatric Dosage

OBJECTIVES

After completing this chapter, the student will be able to:

1. *State the difficulty in defining the appropriate child's dosage for drugs*
2. *State Fried's Rule*
3. *Demonstrate ability to calculate children's dosage using Fried's rule*
4. *State Young's Rule*
5. *Demonstrate ability to calculate children's dosage using Young's rule*
6. *State Clark's Rule*
7. *Demonstrate ability to calculate children's dosage using Clark's rule*
8. *Demonstrate accurate use of West's Nomogram for determining M^2 of skin surface of a child of normal height and weight*
9. *Demonstrate the ability to use West's Nomogram to determine the body surface area of a child not of average height or weight*
10. *Demonstrate the ability to calculate the surface area of a child using the formula*
$$\frac{BSAM^2}{1.7\ M^2} \times Adult\ Dose = Child's\ Dose$$
11. *Demonstrate the ability to convert lbs $\rightleftharpoons$ kg*
12. *Demonstrate the ability to find dosages per body weight (using both kgs of body weight and pounds of body weight).*

Infants and children have special needs in relation to the correct dosage of medication. The growth rate of children for both body weight and height varies greatly from child to child, regardless of age. Many drug reference books do not state pediatric dosages because the variance is so great from one child to the next. The physician prescribes the medication dosage. However, it is the nurse's responsibility to be certain that the child is receiving a therapeutic dose of the drug. In an infant or child, the safe dosage range (the difference between the minimum effective concentration of the drug and the minimum toxic dose) is small. The nurse needs to have some basis on which to judge a safe dosage for the individual child. A small error in dosage calculation could lead to serious, or even fatal, results.

There is no method of drug calculation for children that is completely satisfactory. There are three bases on which children's dosages may be calculated. The formulas used involve age, weight, or body surface area. The formulas based on weight are more accurate than those based on age. Calculations of these dosage formulas are based on the average adult dose, which is the drug dosage to which most ill adults will respond. The difference in the pharmacodynamics of the child's response to the drug differs markedly from that of the adult. There is no substitute for accurate, astute assessment of the child's response to the drug.

Some drug dosages are determined by mg/kg of body weight. However, there are still many drugs on the market that do not take this ratio into consideration. The nurse will find it helpful to know the rules by which childrens' dosages are calculated. Formulas based on the child's age are:

• *Fried's Rule* is used to determine the dosage for infants less than one year of age.

$$\frac{\text{Age of infant in months}}{150} \times \text{adult dose} = \text{Estimated infant's safe dose}$$

(150 - the average adult weight)

The adult dose of a certain drug is 100 mg. Determine the dose for an eight-month-old infant using Fried's Rule.

$$\frac{8 \text{ mo.}}{\underset{3}{\cancel{150}}} \times \overset{2}{\cancel{100}} \text{ mg} = \frac{16}{3} = 5\frac{1}{3} \text{ mg}$$

• *Young's Rule* is used to determine the dose for a child between one and twelve years of age.

$$\frac{\text{Age of child in years}}{\text{Age of child in years} + 12} \times \text{adult dose} = \text{Estimated child's safe dose}$$

The adult dose for a drug is 150 mg. Determine the dose of the drug for a five-year-old child.

$$\frac{5}{5 + 12} \times 150 \text{ mg} = \text{child's dose}$$

$$\frac{5}{17} \times 150 = \frac{750}{17} = 44 \text{ mg}$$

• *Clark's Rule* is used to determine the dosage of children two years of age and older. It is based on the weight of the child and is the most accurate of the three rules, because children vary so much in weight at different ages. This rule is used to determine the approximate correct dose, and is used to check the dose ordered for the child to determine if it is reasonable.

$$\frac{\text{Weight of the child in pounds}}{150} \times \text{adult dose} = \text{Estimated child's safe dose}$$

(average adult weight)

For example, you may wish to know what a reasonable dose of phenobarbital is for a 45 lb child. The adult dose is 60 mg.

$\dfrac{\text{Child's weight}}{\substack{\text{Average adult} \\ \text{weight}}}$ $\dfrac{45 \text{ lbs}}{150 \text{ lbs}}$ × 60 mg = Child's safe dose

$$\frac{\overset{3}{\cancel{45}}}{\underset{10}{\cancel{150}}} \times \frac{6}{\cancel{60}} = 18 \text{ mg}$$

1

BODY SURFACE AREA

Drug dosages for children and adults may be calculated by body surface area (BSA) nomograms and formulas. A nomogram, such as the West Nomogram included on page 104 may be used to determine the BSA from the weight and height of the patient. A formula is then used to determine the drug dose.

To determine BSA, first weigh and measure the child. If the child is normal in height for his body weight, the boxed portion of the nomogram for children of normal height for weight may be used. Place a straight edge (ruler or piece of paper) on the nomogram at the child's weight in pounds. Read the surface area in square meters on the adjacent scale. For example, an average-sized 15 lb child would have a body surface area of 0.36m². Look at this scale carefully and note the changes in the distances between numbers. The scale changes as the numbers get larger; so figure the intervals between the numbers carefully.

If the child is not of normal weight for his height, place a straight edge between the height found on the scale on the left, to the weight found on the scale on the right. Read the surface area where the line intersects with the surface area. The surface area is read in square meters. Thus, if the child weighs 15 kg and is 86 cm tall, the BSA is 0.62m². The next step is to substitute the surface area into the following formula.

$$\frac{\text{Surface area in square meters}}{1.7 \text{ m}^2} \times \text{Adult dose} = \text{Approximate infant or child dose}$$

1.7 m² is the BSA of an average adult

Placing the BSA for the child weighing 15 kg and is 86 cm tall into the formula, calculate an estimated child's dose from an adult dose of 150 mg.

$$\frac{\text{Surface area in square meters}}{1.7} \times \text{Adult dose} = \text{Approximate child's dose}$$

$$\frac{0.62\text{m}^2}{1.7\text{m}^2} \times 150 \text{ mg} = \frac{93}{1.7} = 54.7 \text{ mg Approximate child's dose}$$

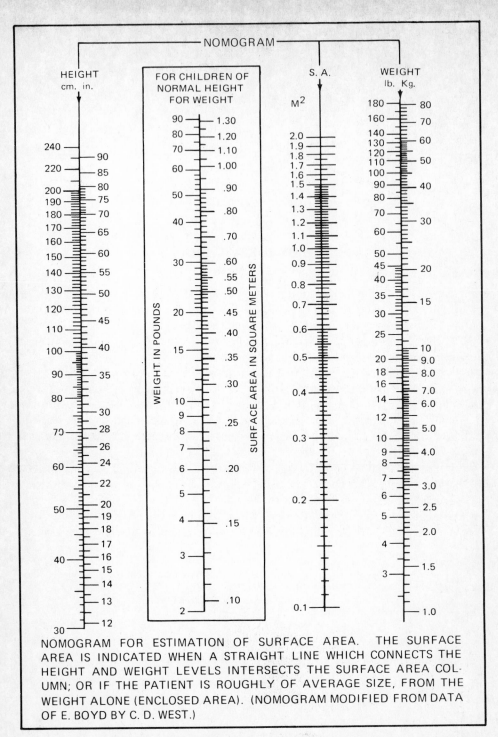

NOMOGRAM

HEIGHT
cm. in.

FOR CHILDREN OF
NORMAL HEIGHT
FOR WEIGHT

S. A.

WEIGHT
lb. Kg.

NOMOGRAM FOR ESTIMATION OF SURFACE AREA. THE SURFACE AREA IS INDICATED WHEN A STRAIGHT LINE WHICH CONNECTS THE HEIGHT AND WEIGHT LEVELS INTERSECTS THE SURFACE AREA COLUMN; OR IF THE PATIENT IS ROUGHLY OF AVERAGE SIZE, FROM THE WEIGHT ALONE (ENCLOSED AREA). (NOMOGRAM MODIFIED FROM DATA OF E. BOYD BY C. D. WEST.)

Fig. 13.1   West Nomogram (for estimation of surface areas). (Nomogram modified from data of E. Boyd by C. D. West. From H. C. Shirkey, "Drug Therapy," in V. C. Vaughan and R. J. McKay (eds.), Nelson Textbook of Pediatrics, 10th ed., W. B. Saunders Company, Philadelphia, 1975, p. 1713)

Use the same formula for the 15 lb child of average height calculate the same drug dosage.

$$\frac{SA\ m^2}{1.7m^2} \times 150\ mg = approximate\ child's\ dose$$

$$\frac{.36m^2}{1.7m^2} \times 150\ mg = \frac{54}{1.7} = 31.76\ mg$$

To Convert kg to lb and lb to kg

The weight must be in kilograms in order to use some nomograms. The West Nomogram uses either pounds or kilograms and centimeters or inches.

To convert pounds to kilograms, simply divide the number of pounds by 2.2.

$$2.2\ lb = 1\ kg$$

To convert from kilograms to pounds, multiply the number of kg by 2.2. Remember a kg is not quite one-half as much as a pound.

Drug Dosage Calculated Per kg or Pound of Body Weight

The drug manufacturers, through research, have determined for many drugs the dosage per kilogram of body weight/day or dose. (Some drugs are calculated per lb/day or dose.)

Simply multiply the child's weight by the suggested dosage to obtain the amount of drug to administer.

● The child's dose of Declomycin is 3–6mg/lb/day in 2–4 divided doses orally. How much drug should a 24 lb child receive per day?

24 lb × 3 mg =   72 mg/day—minimum dose
24 lb × 6 mg = 144 mg/day—maximum dose

How much drug should be given per dose if it is given in four equally divided doses?

$$
\begin{array}{r}
18\ mg/dose \\
4\ \overline{)72\ mg}
\end{array}
$$

$$
\begin{array}{r}
36\ mg/dose \\
4\ \overline{)144}
\end{array}
$$

The dosage range is 18 mg–36 mg/dose.

● The recommended dose of isoniazid (INH) is 10–30 mg/kg/day p.o. Determine the approximate dose for a child weighing 34 kg.

mg/kg = daily dose
34 kg × 10 mg = 340 mg/day
34 kg × 30 mg = 1020 mg/day

The dosage range is 340 mg–1020 mg/day. Divide the daily dose into the recommended doses per day.

The physician will order the drug and dose to be administered to the child. The nurse has the legal responsibility to question any order that does not seem to be correct. By using the appropriate formula, the nurse can determine whether the dose of medication is in the therapeutic range. Remember that a small error in calculation of a child's dose can have serious results.

PROBLEMS: CLARK'S RULE

Using Clark's Rule, determine a safe pediatric dose for the following:

1. The physician ordered aspirin gr iiss for a 40 lb child. The adult dose for aspirin is 300 mg to 600 mg. How much aspirin is safe for a 40 lb child? Is this a safe dose?

2. The physician ordered 25 mg of Meperidine Hcl for a 50 lb child preoperatively. Is this a safe dose? Adult dose is 25 mg to 100 mg.

3. The physician ordered Vistaril 50 mg for a 75 lb boy. The adult dose is 100 mg. Is this a reasonable dose?

4. The physician ordered Bicillin 100,000 U for a 30 lb child. The adult dose is 600,000 U. Is this a reasonable dose?

PROBLEMS: YOUNG'S RULE

5. The average adult dose of a drug is 4 grams. What would be an appropriate dose of the drug for a 10-year-old child?

6. The average adult dose of a drug is 150 mg. What would be an appropriate dose for a six-year-old child?

PROBLEMS: FRIED'S RULE

7. The average adult dose of a drug is 500 mg. What would be an appropriate dose of the drug for a six-month-old infant?

8. The average adult dose of a drug is 250 mg. What would be an appropriate dose of the drug for a three-month-old infant?

PROBLEMS: WEST NOMOGRAM

9.a. Determine the body surface of a child of normal height weighing 22 lbs.

 b. The adult dose of a drug is 4 gm. What is an appropriate dose for the 22 lb child?

10.a. Determine the BSA of a child weighing 40 kg who is 100 cm tall.

 b. The adult dose of Unipen is 500 mg. Determine the child's dose of Unipen.

11. Determine the BSA of a six-pound infant of normal height. The adult dose of gentamicin is 250 mg q 6h.

12. Determine the BSA of a child 80 cm tall, weighing 30 lb. If the adult dose of a drug is 300 mcg, what is the child's dose?

DOSAGE PER WEIGHT

13. A 40 lb child is to receive Unipen. The usual child's dose is 25–50 mg/kg/day in four divided doses. The dosage range for this child will be _____ per day _____ per dose.

14. The child's dose of gentamicin is 3–6 mg/kg/day in divided doses. Determine the dosage range when the infant weighs 6 kg.

15. The child's dose of kanamycin is 7.5–15 mg/kg/day in divided doses. How much drug will a child weighing 45 kg receive?

16. The child's dose of Dilantin is 4–8 mg/kg/day in divided doses. How much drug will a child weighing 60 lbs receive?

ANSWERS: CLARK'S RULE

1. $\dfrac{\text{Child's weight}}{\text{Average adult weight}} \times \dfrac{\text{adult dose}}{} =$ Estimated child's safe dose

$$\dfrac{\overset{4}{\cancel{40}} \text{ lb}}{\underset{\underset{1}{\cancel{15}}}{\cancel{150} \text{ lb}}} \times \overset{20}{\cancel{300}} \text{ mg} = 80 \text{ mg}$$

$$\dfrac{40}{\underset{1}{\cancel{150}}} \times \overset{4}{\cancel{600}} \text{ mg} = 160 \text{ mg}$$

60 mg : 1 gr :: X mg : 2.5 gr
$\qquad\qquad$ X = 150 mg
The dose of aspirin is within the safe range.

2. $\dfrac{\overset{1}{\cancel{50}} \text{ lb}}{\underset{3}{\cancel{150} \text{ lb}}} \times 25 \text{ mg.} = \dfrac{25}{3} = 8\ 1/3 \text{ mg}$

$$\dfrac{\overset{1}{\cancel{50}} \text{ lb}}{\underset{3}{\cancel{150} \text{ lb}}} \times 100 \text{ mg.} = \dfrac{100}{3} = 33.3 \text{ mg}$$

The estimated range for a 50 lb child is 8.3 mg to 33.3 mg. The order is within this range.

3. $\dfrac{75 \text{ lb}}{150 \text{ lb}} \times 100 \text{ mg} = \dfrac{150}{3} = 50 \text{ mg}$ $\qquad$ *The dose is safe.*

4. $\dfrac{30}{\underset{1}{\cancel{150}}} \times \overset{4000}{\cancel{600,000}} \text{ U} = 120,000 \text{ Units}$ $\qquad$ *The dose is safe.*

ANSWERS: YOUNG'S RULE

5. $\dfrac{\text{Age of child}}{\text{Age of child } + 12} \times \text{Adult dose} = \text{Estimated child's dose}$

$\dfrac{10}{10 + 12} \times 4 \text{ gm} = \dfrac{40}{22} = 1.8 \text{ gm}$

or

$\dfrac{10}{10 + 12} \times 400 \text{ mg} = \dfrac{4000}{22} = 181.8 \text{ mg}$

6. $\dfrac{6}{6 + 12} \times 150 \text{ mg} = \dfrac{900}{18} = 50 \text{ mg}$

ANSWERS: FRIED'S RULE

7. $\dfrac{\text{age in months}}{150 \text{ average adult weight}} \times \text{Adult dose} = \text{Estimated infant dose}$

$\dfrac{6 \text{ mo}}{150 \text{ lb}} \times 500 \text{ mg} = \dfrac{3000}{150} = 20 \text{ mg}$

8. $\dfrac{\text{age in months}}{150} \times \text{Adult dose} = \text{Estimated infant dose}$

$\dfrac{3 \text{ mo}}{150 \text{ lb}} \times 250 \text{ mg} = \dfrac{750}{150} = 5 \text{ mg}$

ANSWERS: CALCULATING DOSAGE USING BODY SURFACE AREA

9. a. Body surface area: 0.47 m^2

b. $\dfrac{\text{surface area m}^2}{1.7} \times \text{A.D.} = \text{CD}$

$\dfrac{0.47 \text{ m}^2}{1.7 \text{ m}^2} \times 4 \text{ gm} = \dfrac{1.88}{1.7} = 1.1 \text{ gm}$

10. a. 1.14 m^2

$\dfrac{1.14 \text{ m}^2}{1.7 \text{ m}^2} \times 500 \text{ mg} = \dfrac{570}{1.7} = 335 \text{ mg}$

11. a. 0.2 m²

   b. $\dfrac{0.2 \text{ m}^2}{1.7 \text{ m}^2} \times 250 \text{ mg} = \dfrac{50}{1.7} = 29.4 \text{ mg}$

12. a. 0.58 m²

   b. $\dfrac{0.58 \text{ m}^2}{1.7 \text{ m}^2} \times 300 \text{ mcg} = \dfrac{174}{1.7} = 102.35 \text{ mcg}$

ANSWERS: DOSAGE PER WEIGHT

13. 40 lb child

$$2.2 \overline{)40 \text{ lb.}}^{\,18 \text{ kg}}$$

   18 kg × 25 mg = 450 mg/day   112.5 mg/dose
   18 kg × 50 mg = 900 mg/day   225 mg/dose
   Range 450 mg–900 mg/day   *112.5 mg–225 mg/dose*

14. 6 kg × 3 mg = 18 mg/day
   6 kg × 6 mg = 36 mg/day
   Range 18 mg–36 mg/day

15. 45 kg × 7.5 mg = 337.5 mg/day
   45 kg × 15 mg = 675 mg/day
   337.5–675 mg/day
   84 mg–168.7 mg/dose

16. a. $2.2 \overline{)60 \text{ lb}}^{\,27.27 \text{ kg}}$

   27 kg × 4 mg = 108 mg/day

14 Conversion of Temperature Between Fahrenheit and Celsius

OBJECTIVES

After completing this chapter, the student will be able to:

1. *Convert a temperature from Fahrenheit to Celsius, using a conversion formula*
2. *Convert a temperature from Celsius to Fahrenheit, using a conversion formula.*

The temperature of a patient is one of the physiologic indications of the patient's state of health. A temperature elevation may be an indication that a patient needs antibiotic therapy and/or the patient may need a drug to lower the temperature. The nurse must keep an accurate record of the patient's temperature. The nurse should be able to convert from Celsius to Fahrenheit temperature and vice versa.

Originally the term centigrade was used in place of Celsius. Celsius is the metric term and so we will use this term. Five degrees on the Celsius scale equals nine degrees on the Fahrenheit scale. Therefore the fractions 5/9 and 9/5 are used to convert temperatures from one scale to the other. These fractions indicate the relationship of one scale to the other.

There are a number of formulas that may be used for temperature conversion. I prefer a single formula to convert either way. I will also give a formula to convert from Fahrenheit to Celsius and a formula to convert from Celsius to Fahrenheit. Choose the method that you find easiest.

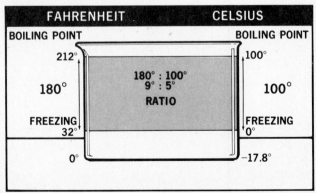

Figure 14.1

Use this formula for conversion to either scale.

$$\frac{9}{5}C = F - 32$$

Convert 100° F to C

$$\frac{9}{5}C = F - 32$$

$$\frac{9}{5}C = 100 - 32$$

$$\frac{9}{5}C = 68$$

$$\frac{9}{5} \div \frac{9}{5}C = 68 \div \frac{9}{5}$$

$$\frac{\cancel{9}}{\cancel{5}} \times \frac{\cancel{5}}{\cancel{9}}C = 68 \times \frac{5}{9}$$

$$C = \frac{340}{9}$$

$$C = 37.77 \text{ or } 37.8°$$

Convert 37.8° C to F

$$\frac{9}{5}C = F - 32$$

$$\frac{9}{5} \cdot 37.8 = F - 32$$

$$\frac{340.2}{5} = F - 32$$

$$68 + 32 = F - 32 + 32$$

$$100° = F$$

1. To convert from Fahrenheit to Celsius temperature:

   Subtract 32° from the Fahrenheit temperature
   Multiply the result by 5/9
   C = (F − 32) × 5/9

Remember the difference in the freezing point on the 2 scales is 32° and the ratio between the scales is 5:9 or 5/9

Example: Convert 100° F to C

$$C = (F-32) \times 5/9$$
$$C = (100°-32) \times 5/9$$
$$C = 68 \times 5/9$$
$$C = \frac{340}{9}$$
$$C = 37.77 \text{ or } 37.8°$$

2. To convert from Celsius to Fahrenheit temperature:

   Multiply the Celsius temperature by 9/5 and add 32°

   F = (9/5 C) + 32

Example: Convert 37.8°C to F

$$F = (9/5 \ \ C) + 32$$
$$F = (9/5 \times 37.8) + 32$$
$$F = 68.04 + 32$$
$$F = 100°$$

PROBLEMS: TEMPERATURE CONVERSION

Convert the following temperatures as indicated. Give answers in decimal form rounded off to the nearest tenth of a degree. Show your work.

1. 37°C _____ F

2. 38.9°C _____ F

3. 36.7°C _____ F

4. 101°F _____ C

5. 97°F _____ C

6. 104°F _____ C

ANSWERS: TEMPERATURE CONVERSION

1) $9/5C = F - 32$
   $9/5 (37) = F - 32$
   $32 + 66.6 = F. - 32 + 32$
   $98.6° = F$

   $37°C = \underline{98.6\ F.}$
   $F = (9/5\ C) + 32°$
   $F = (9/5 \times 37°) + 32°$
   $F = \dfrac{333}{5} + 32°$
   $F = 98.6°$

2) $9/5C = F - 32$
   $9/5 (38.9) = F - 32$
   $32 + 70.02 = F - 32 + 32$
   $102.02 = F$
   $102° = F$

   $38.9°C = \underline{102°F.}$
   $F = (9/5 \times 38.9) + 32$
   $F = \dfrac{(350.1)}{5} + 32$
   $F = 70 + 32$
   $F = 102°$

3) $9/5C = F - 32$
   $9/5 (36.7) = F - 32$
   $32 + \dfrac{330.3}{5} = F - 32 + 32$
   $32 + 66.06 = F$
   $98.06 = F$
   $98° = F$

   $36.7°C = \underline{98°F.}$
   $F = (9/5 \times 36.7) + 32$
   $F = \dfrac{(330.3)}{5} + 32$
   $F = 66 + 32$
   $F = 98.06$
   $F = 98°$

4) $9/5C = (F - 32)$
$9/5C = (101 - 32)$
$9/5C = 69$
$9/5 \div 9/5\ C = 69 \div 9/5$
$9/5 \times 5/9\ C = 69 \times 5/9 = \dfrac{345}{9}$
$C = 38.3°$

$101°F = \underline{38.3°C.}$
$C = (F - 32°) \times 5/9$
$C = (101° - 32°) \times 5/9$
$C = 69 \times 5/9$
$C = \dfrac{345}{9}$
$C = 38.3°$

5) $9/5C = F - 32$
$9/5C = 97° - 32$
$9/5 \div 9/5\ C = 65 \div 9/5$
$C = 65 \times 5/9 = \dfrac{325}{9}$
$C = 36.1°$

$97°F = \underline{36.1°C.}$
$C = (97° - 32) \times 5/9$
$C = 65 \times 5/9$
$C = \dfrac{325}{9}$
$C = 36.1°$

6) $9/5C = F - 32$
$9/5C = 104° - 32$
$9/5 \div 9/5C = 72 \div 9/5$
$9/5 \times 5/9C = 72 \times 5/9$
$C = \dfrac{360}{9}$
$C = 40°$

$104°F = \underline{40°C.}$
$C = (104° - 32) \times 5/9$
$C = 72 \times 5/9$
$C = \dfrac{360}{9}$
$C = 40°$

15   Computerization of Drug Records

OBJECTIVES

After completing this chapter, the student will be able to:

1. *Recognize the components of a computer printout*
2. *Read the time from the twenty-four-hour clock*
3. *Write the time of day using the twenty-four-hour clock*

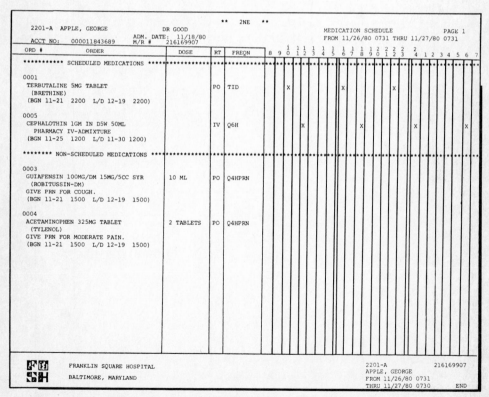

Figure 15.1

To simplify the enormous job of record keeping, hospital pharmacies are converting to a computerized system. As the medication orders are sent to the pharmacy, the pharmacist will add the new drugs to the computer listing and delete the drugs that have been discontinued. A medication sheet containing all current drugs ordered for the patient will be sent to the patient's nursing unit each day. This system will save the nursing unit time that was formerly spent transcribing medication orders to a Kardex and/or medication cards.

Included on the printout sheet will be all of the patient's medications, dose, frequency of administration, route, and times of administration. The computerized medication sheet will have the advantages of containing more detailed information and greater consistency and accuracy than the systems currently in use in most hospitals.

Look at the computer printout sheet, page 115.

The top of the sheet contains the patient's name, hospital number, and other information pertinent to identification, the inclusive date, and the time period which the sheet represents.

In the left hand column, ORD# is the number of the physician's order. Each order written will have a sequenced number (activity orders, laboratory tests, diet, medications, etc.) making it easier to refer back to the chart and the medication order in question.

Under "order," the drug may be listed by both generic and proprietary name; the time the medication was started; and the time of the last dose to be given.

						TIMES
						1 1 1 1 1
Order #	*Order*	*Dose*	*Rt*	*Freqn*		*8 9 0 1 2 3 4*
0001	Terbutaline	5 mg	Po	Tid		X
	BGN (Begin)	11/21 (Date)	2200 (Time)	L/D (Last dose)	12/19 (Date)	2200 (time)

Each hospital will decide on the format to be used by that hospital.

The nurse must learn to tell time by the twenty-four-hour clock in order to use these medication sheets.

Study the twenty-four-hour clock and complete the work sheets.

THE TWENTY-FOUR-HOUR CLOCK

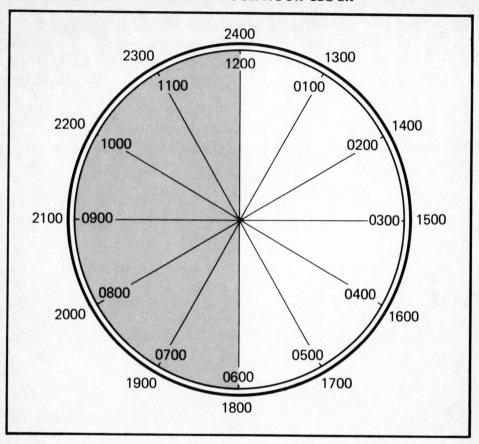

Figure 15.2   The Twenty-Four-Hour Clock.

The numbers inside the clock represent the hours from 1 AM until 12 noon. The numbers on the outside of the clock represent the time from 1 PM until midnight.

To tell time read the numbers, as 0100, or zero 100 hours, 1 AM; 0200 hours, for 2 AM; and so on around the clock until 12 noon, 1200 hours. 1 PM is 1300 hours, 2 PM is 1400 hours and finally 12 midnight is 2400. One twenty-five PM would be 1325 hours, or thirteen hundred twenty-five hours.

The time from 12 midnight to 1 AM is stated, 0001, 0002, 0005, 0010, 0015, 0030, 0045, etc. Minutes only are stated.

PROBLEMS: THE TWENTY-FOUR-HOUR CLOCK

Given the traditional clock time, state the time according to the twenty-four-hour clock.

Exercise I

1. 9 PM _____   6. 10:25 AM _____

2. 4 AM _____   7. 3:30 PM _____

3. 4:05 PM _____   8. 2 AM _____

4. 6:30 AM _____   9. 10 PM _____

5. 8:15 PM _____   10. 12 Midnight _____

Exercise II

Given the time using the twenty-four-hour clock, state the time according to the traditional clock.

1. 1315 hours _____   6. 0230 hours _____

2. 0345 hours _____   7. 0400 hours _____

3. 0620 hours _____   8. 1645 hours _____

4. 2015 hours _____   9. 1010 hours _____

5. 2325 hours _____   10. 2215 hours _____

ANSWERS: THE TWENTY-FOUR-HOUR CLOCK

Given the traditional clock time, state the time according to the twenty-four-hour clock.

Exercise I

1. 9 PM <u>2100 twenty one hundred hours</u>

6. 10:25 AM <u>1025 ten twenty-five hours</u>

2. 4 AM <u>0400 zero four hundred hours</u>

7. 3:30 PM <u>1530 fifteen hundred thirty hours</u>

3. 4:05 PM <u>1605 sixteen 0 five hours</u>

8. 2 AM <u>0200 zero two hundred hours</u>

4. 6:30 AM <u>0630 zero six thirty hours</u>

9. 10 PM <u>2200 twenty two hundred hours</u>

5. 8:15 PM <u>2015 twenty fifteen hours</u>

10. 12 Midnight <u>2400 twenty four hundred hours</u>

118
Drug Dosages and Solutions Workbook

Exercise II

Given the time using the twenty-four-hour clock, state the time according to the traditional clock.

1. 1315 hours <u>1:15 PM</u>

2. 0345 hours <u>3:45 AM</u>

3. 0620 hours <u>6:20 AM</u>

4. 2015 hours <u>8:15 PM</u>

5. 2325 hours <u>11:25 PM</u>

6. 0230 hours <u>2:30 AM</u>

7. 0400 hours <u>4:00 AM</u>

8. 1645 hours <u>4:45 PM</u>

9. 1010 hours <u>10:10 AM</u>

10. 2215 hours <u>10:15 PM</u>

Practice Problems

1. Give 750 mg of a drug. Label reads 0.25 gm tablets.

2. Give ASA (aspirin) 1.5 gm On hand 0.3 gm tablets.

3. Give ammonium chloride 2 gm Stock bottle 0.2 gm/ml.

4. Give 20,000 U from a bottle labeled 100,000 U/10 ml.

5. Give 200,000 U from a bottle labeled 1,000,000 U/10 ml.

6. Give 2 gm of a drug from a 20% solution. Label reads 20 gm/100 ml.

7. Give 2 gm of a drug from a 20% solution. Label reads 0.2 gm/ml.

8. The label on a stock bottle reads 0.5 mg/cc. The order reads give 0.08 mg.

9. The label on the stock bottle reads 0.5 mg/ml. The order reads give 0.01 mg.

10. The label on the stock bottle reads 100 mg in 2 ml. The order reads give 25 mg.

Section B

Read all problems carefully. Show all work. Label correctly.

1. Prepare 8 gm of $MgSO_4$ for IM administration from a 50% solution.
   Give _____

2. The doctor orders aspirin gr viiss. The tablets on hand are gr v tablets.

3. Give Kaon Elixir 15 mEq. Available 20 mEq per 30 ml. Give _____

4. Give Ampicillin 0.15 gm P.O. from a stock bottled labeled 500 mg/5 ml.
   Give _____

5. Using Clark's Rule, determine the child's dose. The adult dose of phenobarbital is 80 mg. What is the dose for a child weighing 45 lb?

6. Prepare 500 ml of 10% glycerin solution from liquid glycerin.
   Drug _____
   Solvent _____

7. Give Keflin 750 mg. Vial is labeled 0.5 gm in 2.2 ml. Give _____

8. You have scored tablets of Digoxin labeled 0.25 mg. Give 0.000125 gm.

9. A drug is labeled gr $\frac{1}{100}$ in 15 m. Give gr $\frac{1}{150}$ _____

10. The doctor has ordered 1000 ml of D$_5$W to run IV for 8 hours. The drop factor is 10 gtts/ml. At what rate should this IV run? _____

11. The doctor orders 62 Units of NPH insulin to be given before breakfast. Insulin on hand 100-U/ml. (U-100) How would you prepare this dose using an insulin syringe?

12. 1 ml   _____ M

    ℥ II   _____ ℨ

    3 tbsp   _____ ounce

    1 pt   _____ L

    4000 ml   _____ gal

13. Give 300,000 U of crystalline penicillin IM. In the medicine room you find a bottle of 1,000,000 U of crystalline penicillin in dry form. Add 3.6 ml of diluent and shake. Each ml contains 500,000 U after reconstitution. The nurse will give _____

14. Give 750 mg of Prostaphlin IM. In the medicine room you have a 2 gm bottle of Prostaphin. Add 5.7 ml of distilled water to the vial. After mixing each 1.5 ml will contain 500 mg. The nurse will give _____

15
&
16. Your patient is going to O.R. You must give Demerol 60 mg and Atropine 0.3 mg IM preoperatively. On hand you have a 2 ml ampule of Demerol containing 50 mg/ml. Give _____ of Demerol. You have Atropine 1 mg/1 cc. Give _____ Atropine.

17. Convert the following temperatures.

     104°F = _____ C

     35°C   = _____ F

18. The doctor orders gr 1/60 of a drug. On hand tab. gr 1/80. Give _____

19. Give Elix. Phenobarbital 6 mg from a stock bottle containing 20 mg/5 cc. Give _____

ANSWERS: SECTION A

1. 3 tab.

2. 5 tab.

3. 10 ml

4. 2 ml

5. 2 ml

6. 10 ml

7. 10 ml

8. 0.16 ml

9. 0.02 ml

10. 0.5 ml

ANSWERS: SECTION B

1. 16 ml

2. 1.5 tab.

3. 22.5 ml

4. 1.5 ml

5. 24 mg = CD

6. 50 ml (Drug)   450 ml (Solvent)

7. 3.3 ml

8. 0.5 tab. ½ tab.

9. 0.66 ml or ℥ ×

10. 21 gtts/min

11. Using a U-100 syringe, draw up U-100 N.P.H. insulin to the 62 Unit mark.

12. 15-16 M
    16 ʒ
    1½ ounce
    0.5 L
    1 gal

13. 0.6 ml

14. 2.25 ml

15
&
16. 1.2 ml of Demerol   0.3 ml Atropine

17. 40°C   95°F

18. 1.33 or 1⅓ tab.

19. 1.5 ml of Elix. Phenobarbital

PRACTICE TEST

Read all problems carefully. Work accurately. Label each answer.

1. The doctor orders 0.375 mg of digoxin.
   The tablets on hand are 0.25 mg strength.
   The nurse must give _____

2. The doctor orders Thiosulfil 1 gm.
   The tablets on hand are 250 mg.
   The nurse must give _____

3. Convert the following temperatures:
   (a) 50°F _____ C
   (b) 72°C _____ F

4. The doctor orders 10 gm of chloral hydrate.
   Available is a vial containing a 25% solution.
   The nurse will give _____

5. The doctor orders 3000 ml of D_5 RL to be given in 24 hours. The drop factor is 20 gtts/ml. How many drops per minute should this IV run?

6. The doctor orders liver extract 80 mcg (micrograms)
   The vial available is labeled 200 mcg per 10 ml.
   The nurse must give _____

7. The doctor orders calcium gluceptate 540 mg to be added to IV fluids. You have available 5 ml ampules containing 90 mg of calcium gluceptate.
The nurse must add _____

8. The nurse must give potassium chloride 40 mEq. She has a Unit dose bottle containing 20 mEq per 10 ml.
The nurse must give _____

9. The nurse must give Polycillin 1 gm p.o. She has available a 100 ml bottle of Polycillin for oral suspension. To prepare add a total of 81 ml water. Shake well. This provides 100 ml of suspension. Each 5 ml contains Polycillin equivalent to 250 mg.
The nurse must give _____

10. From a vial labeled Heparin 20,000 Units per ml give 15,000 Units of Heparin.
Give: _____

11. Give penicillin 1,500,000 Units from a solution labeled 3,000,000 Units per 5 ml.
The nurse must give _____

12. Give Dilaudid gr $\frac{1}{6}$ from gr $\frac{1}{3}$ tablets
The nurse must give _____

13. Give Atropine Sulphate gr $\frac{1}{200}$

Tablets available gr $\frac{1}{300}$

The nurse must give _____

14. How will you make 1 L or 35% lysol solution? Lysol is a pure liquid drug.
Drug _____
Solvent _____

15. Using Clark's Rule, what is the average dose for a child weighing 60 pounds if an adult dose of Terramycin is 100 mg?

_____

16. The adult dose is 300,000 Units of penicillin. Using Clark's Rule, how much penicillin will a 50 lb child receive?

_____

17. Make 250 ml of physiologic salt solution (0.9%). Use salt crystals.
Drug _____
Solvent _____

18. How would you prepare 85 Units of U-100 NPH insulin? Use an insulin syringe.

_____

19. 15 grains _____ gm
4 drams _____ oz
1 qt. _____ ml
½ oz. _____ tbsp
4000 ml. _____ gal

20. 1 ml _____ minims
1 pt. O i _____ ml
1 tsp. _____ ℥ _____ ml
30 ml. _____ tablespoons

```
┌─────────────────────────────────────────────┐  ┌──────────────────────────────┐
│          ┌─────────────────┐                │  │ NAME                         │
│          │ 5,000,000 Units │                │  │    Will Johnson              │
│          └─────────────────┘                │  │ ROOM  START  STOP            │
│   PENICILLIN G POTASSIUM FOR INJECTION      │  │  201  12-15-80 12-25         │
│           USP (BUFFERED)                    │  │ DRUG                         │
│       Preparation of Solution               │  │  Potassium Penicillin        │
│       Add          Concentration of         │  │ DOSE                         │
│       Diluent          Solution             │  │   400,000 Units              │
│                                             │  │ TIME  8 - 2 - 8 - 2          │
│       18 ml...........250,000 units/ml      │  └──────────────────────────────┘
│        8 ml...........500,000 units/ml      │
│        3 ml.........1,000,000 units/ml      │
└─────────────────────────────────────────────┘
```

21. Give 400,000 Units Potassium Penicillin G.
    a. How much diluent must you add to make the strength needed? _____
    b. What is the dosage strength of the solution you mixed? _____
    c. How much Potassium Penicillin G does this vial contain? _____
    d. Compute dosage to be given.

22. Using Freid's rule determine the dosage for an 11-month-old infant for a drug when the adult dose is 240 mg.

23. Using Young's rule determine the safe dose of a medication for a 7-year-old child. The adult dose is 30 mg.

24. The recommended dose of streptomycin for a premature infant is 15 to 30 mg/kg/day. What is the recommended dosage range for a 4 lb infant?

25. Using West's Nomogram (page 104) determine the body surface area for a child weighing 33 lb with a height of 34 inches.
    Using the body surface area formula calculate the dosage of a drug if the adult dose is 75 mg.

26. Look at the computer printout sheet (Page 115). State in traditional time the hours Mr. Apple is to receive Terbutaline.

27. An intravenous medication has been reconstituted into 60 ml of solution. The medication is to be administered in 30 minutes. The drop factor is 20 gtt/ml. How many drops per minute should this IV infuse?

28. The doctor ordered 20 gm of Mg SO$_4$ to be added to 1000 ml of D$_5$W. Infuse at 1.5 gm/hour. The drop factor is 13 gtt/ml. How much fluid is to be infused in 1 hr? How many gtts/min should this IV infuse?

29. Prepare 500 ml of a 0.5% solution from a 2% solution.
    Solute _____
    Solvent _____

30. If 375 ml of drug was used to prepare 1500 ml of solution, what is the percentage strength of this solution?

31. Convert
     65 lb = _____ kg
     225 lb = _____ kg
     75 kg = _____ lb
     33 kg = _____ lb
     3.8 kg = _____ lb

ANSWERS: PRACTICE TEST

1. $\dfrac{0.375 \text{ mg}}{0.25 \text{ mg}} \times 1 \text{ tab} = 1\ 1/2$ tablets of digoxin 0.25 mg

2. 1 gm = 1000 mg

   250 mg: 1 tab :: 1000 mg: X tab
   250 X = 1000
        X = 4 tablets of 250 mg Thiosulfil

3. (a) $C = (F-32) \times 5/9$

   $C = (50-32) \times 5/9$

   $$C = \overset{2}{\cancel{18}} \times \frac{5}{\underset{1}{\cancel{9}}}$$

   $C = 10°$

(b) $F = (9/5 \times C) + 32$

   $F = (9/5) \times 72) + 32$

   $$F = \frac{648.0}{5} + 32$$

   $F = 129.6 + 32$

   $F = 161.6$

4. $\dfrac{25\ gm}{100\ ml} : \dfrac{10\ gm}{X\ ml}$

   $25\ X = 1000$

   $X = 40$ ml of chloral hydrate

5.

$$\begin{array}{r} 125\ ml. \\ 24\ \overline{)3000\ ml.} \\ \underline{24} \\ 60 \\ \underline{48} \\ 120 \\ \underline{120} \end{array}$$

= 1 hr volume

= 24 hr volume

$$\frac{20\ gtts/ml}{60\ min} \times 125\ ml = gtts/min$$

$$\frac{\overset{1}{\cancel{20}}}{\underset{3}{\cancel{60}}} \times 125 = \frac{125}{3} = 42\ gtts/min\ to\ run\ IV$$

6. $\dfrac{80\ mcg}{200\ mcg} \times 10\ ml = \dfrac{\overset{8}{\cancel{80}}\ mcg}{\underset{\underset{2}{20}}{\cancel{200}}\ mcg} \times \overset{1}{\cancel{10}}\ ml = \dfrac{8}{2} = 4\ ml$

7. 90 mg: 5 ml :: 540 mg: $\times$ ml

   $90\ X = 2700$

   $X = 30$ ml of calcium gluceptate or use 6 ampules

   $$90\ mg\ \overline{)540\ mg}^{\ \ 6\ \ amps}$$

8. $\dfrac{\overset{2}{\cancel{40}}\ mEq}{\underset{1}{\cancel{20}}\ mEq} \times 10\ ml = 20\ ml\ of\ KCl$

9. 250 mg : 5 ml :: 1000 mg : X ml

   $250\ X = 5000$

   $X = 20$ ml of Polycillin

10. $\dfrac{\overset{3}{\cancel{15,000}}}{\underset{4}{\cancel{20,000}}} \times 1\ ml = \dfrac{3}{4}$ $4\ \overline{)3.00}\ ^{0.75}$ ml of Heparin

11. 3,000,000 U : 5 ml :: 1,500,000 U : X ml

$$3,000,000\ X = 7,500,000$$
$$X = \dfrac{75\cancel{00000}}{30\cancel{00000}} = 30\ \overline{)75.0}\ ^{2.5} \qquad X = 2.5\ ml\ of\ penicillin$$
$$\underline{60}$$
$$150$$
$$\underline{150}$$

12. $\dfrac{1/6}{1/3} \times 1\ tab = X$

$$\dfrac{1}{6} \div \dfrac{1}{3} \times 1 = X$$

$$\dfrac{1}{\underset{2}{\cancel{6}}} \times \dfrac{\overset{1}{\cancel{3}}}{1} \times 1 = 1/2\ tab\ \textbf{(Dilaudid)}$$

13. $\dfrac{1}{300} : 1\ tab :: \dfrac{1}{200} : X\ tab$

$$\dfrac{1}{300}\ X = \dfrac{1}{200}$$

$$\dfrac{1}{300} \div \dfrac{1}{300}\ X = \dfrac{1}{200} \div \dfrac{1}{300}$$

$$\dfrac{1}{\cancel{300}} \times \dfrac{\cancel{300}}{1}\ X = \dfrac{1}{\underset{2}{\cancel{200}}} \times \dfrac{\overset{3}{\cancel{300}}}{1}$$

$$X = \dfrac{3}{2} = 1\ 1/2\ tab\ \textbf{(Atropine Sulfate)}$$

14. $\dfrac{35}{\underset{1}{\cancel{100}}} \times \overset{10}{\cancel{1000}}\ ml = 350\ ml\ of\ lysol\ solution = Drug$

$$\begin{aligned}
&1000\ ml\\
-&\ 350\ ml\\
\hline
&650\ ml
\end{aligned}$$ of solvent to be added to drug to make 1000 ml of solution

15. $\dfrac{\overset{20}{\cancel{60}}}{\cancel{150}} \times \overset{2}{\cancel{100}}$ mg = Child's dose

 20 × 2 = 40 mg of Terramycin may be given to a 60 lb child

16. $\dfrac{\overset{50}{\cancel{150}}}{\underset{1}{\cancel{150}}} \times \overset{2000}{\cancel{300,000}}$ U = C.D.

 50 × 2000 = 100,000 U of Penicillin may be given to a 50 lb child

17. $\dfrac{0.9 \text{ gm}}{100 \text{ ml}} :: \dfrac{X \text{ gm}}{250 \text{ ml}}$ OR 0.9 gm : 100 ml :: X gm : 250 ml

 100 X = 225.0
 X = 2.25 gm of salt = drug

Solvent - Place 2.25 gm of salt in container and add enough water to equal 250 ml.

18. Using a U-100 syringe, draw up Lente U-100 insulin to the 85 U mark on the syringe.

19. 15 grains <u>1</u> gm
 4 drams <u>1/2</u> oz
 1 qt <u>1000</u> ml
 1/2 oz <u>1</u> tbsp
 4000 ml <u>1</u> gal

20. 1 ml <u>15</u> minims
 1 pt <u>500</u> ml
 1 teaspoon <u>1ζ 4-5</u> ml
 30 ml <u>2</u> tablespoons

21. a. 8 ml
 b. 500,000/ml
 c. 5,000,000 U
 d. 0.8 ml

 $\dfrac{\overset{4}{\cancel{400,000}} \text{ U}}{\underset{5}{\cancel{500,000}} \text{ U}} \times 1 \text{ ml} = \dfrac{4}{5} = 0.8$ ml

22. $\dfrac{\text{age of infant in months}}{150} \times$ Adult dose = Child's dose

$$\frac{11 \text{ months}}{\cancel{150} \text{ lbs}} \times \cancel{240}^{\,24}\text{mg} = \frac{264}{15} = 17.6\text{mg}$$
$$\phantom{\frac{11}{150}}^{15}$$

23. $\dfrac{\text{age of child in years}}{\text{age of child in years} + 12} \times \text{adult dose} = \text{Child's dose}$

$$\frac{7 \text{ yr}}{7 \text{ yr} + 12} \times 30\text{mg} = \frac{7}{19} \times 30 = \frac{210}{19} = 11\text{mg}$$

24. $4 \text{ lb} \div 2.2 = 1.8\text{kg}$
    $15\text{mg} \times 1.8\text{kg} = 27\text{mg/day}$
    $30\text{mg} \times 1.8\text{kg} = 54\text{mg/day}$
    The dosage range of streptomycin for a 4 lb infant is 27mg to 54mg per day

25. $0.61\text{m}^2 = \text{BSA}$

$$\frac{\text{surface area m}^2}{1.7 \text{ m}^2} \times \text{adult dose} = \text{child's dose}$$

$$\frac{0.61\text{m}^2}{1.7\text{m}^2} \times 75\text{mg} = \frac{45.75}{1.7} = 26.9\text{mg}$$

26. 10 A.M.   4 P.M.   10 P.M.

27. $\dfrac{20 \text{ gtt/ml}}{30 \text{ min}} \times 60\text{ml} = 40\text{gtts/min}$

28. $\dfrac{D}{H} \times V = \text{Amt. to be infused per hour}$

$$\frac{1.5\text{gm}}{\cancel{20}\text{gm}} \times 1000\text{ml}^{\,50} = 75 \text{ ml/hr needed to administer 1.5 gm of MgSO}_4\text{/hr}$$
$$\phantom{\frac{1.5}{20}}^{1}$$

OR

20gm : 1000ml :: 1.5gm : X ml
    20 X = 1500
       X = 75ml/hr

$$\frac{\text{Drop factor}}{60 \text{ min}} \times 1 \text{ hr Vol} = \text{gtt/min}$$

$$\frac{13 \text{ gtt/ml}}{\cancel{60} \text{ min}} \times \cancel{75}\,\text{ml} = \frac{195}{12} = 16.25 = 16 \text{ gtt/min rate IV to infuse}$$
$$\phantom{\frac{13}{60}}_{12}^{\ 15}$$

29. 0.5ml : 2ml :: X ml : 500 ml

   2 X = 250

   X = 125 ml of 2% solution needed to make 500 ml of a 0.5% solution

OR

$$\frac{0.5 \text{ ml.}}{2 \text{ ml}} \times 500 \text{ ml} = 125 \text{ ml}$$

$$
\begin{array}{r}
500 \text{ ml}\ \ \text{solution} \\
- 125 \text{ ml}\ \ \text{solute} \\
\hline
375 \text{ ml}\ \ \text{solvent}
\end{array}
$$

30. X ml : 100 ml :: 375 ml : 1500 ml

   1500 X = 37500

   X = 25 ml $\dfrac{25\text{ml}}{100\text{ml}}$ = 25% solution

31.   65 lb = 29.55 kg
     225 lb = 102.27 kg
     75 kg = 165 lb
     33 kg = 72.6 lb
     3.8 kg = 8.36 lb